Conducting Effective Conferences
with Parents of Children with Disabilities

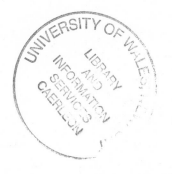

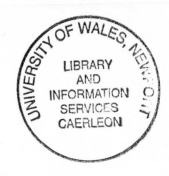
Conducting Effective Conferences with Parents of Children with Disabilities

A Guide for Teachers

Milton Seligman

THE GUILFORD PRESS
New York   London

© 2000 The Guilford Press
A Division of Guilford Publications, Inc.
72 Spring Street, New York, NY 10012
www.guilford.com

Printed in the United States of America

This book is printed on acid-free paper.

Last digit is print number: 9 8 7 6 5 4 3 2 1

Library of Congress Cataloging-in-Publication Data

Seligman, Milton, 1937–
    Conducting effective conferences with parents of children with
    disabilities : a guide for teachers / Milton Seligman.
        p. cm.
    Includes bibliographical references (p.) and index.
    ISBN 1-57230-537-1 (pbk.)—ISBN 1-57230-553-3 (hc.)
    1. Handicapped children—Education. 2. Parents of handicapped
    children—Counseling of. 3. Parent–teacher conferences. I. Title.

LC4019.S385 2000
371.103—dc21   99-056731
                                                                  CIP

In memory of Beth Cohen

And to her pal, Lori

About the Author

Milton Seligman, PhD, is Professor and Chair of the Counseling Psychology Program at the University of Pittsburgh. He has taught courses in Individual and Group Psychotherapy, Clinical Supervision, and Disability and the Family, and has published and lectured widely on the subject of disability and the family. Dr. Seligman also consults in the area of disability and rehabilitation and maintains a part-time private practice.

He has two daughters in their late 20s, one of whom has a disability. Despite her disability, Dr. Seligman's daughter is relatively independent and is employed in a part-time position in a children's museum. She also volunteers for a variety of disability and non-disability-related causes.

Preface

In the mid- to late 1970s I taught a course at the University of Pittsburgh in how to engage and collaborate with parents of children with disabilities. At that time, when reforms in special education were just beginning, there were few such courses on parent–teacher conferences and little written on this topic. Back then, children with special needs were largely placed into special education classes based on the child's disability, and special education teachers conducted conferences with parents. Unlike present-day practice, these conferences focused mostly on the child's education, not on ancillary services such as speech therapy, assistive technology, and occupational therapy.

Fortunately, much has changed since the mid-1970s. Today full inclusion, rather than segregation and limited collaboration with parents, is the norm, whereas in the 1970s there was no inclusion as we know it today. Public Law 94-142, the Education for All Handicapped Children Act passed in 1975, was in its infancy. Regular schoolteachers were not routine participants in Individualized Education Program (IEP) conferences. Their involvement with children who had special needs and their parents was just beginning, as the concept of integration was being both implemented and debated by parents and educators. The central issue being debated was the wisdom of educating regular and special education children together. Although echoes of the debate are still heard today, the concept of inclusion now has a firm foothold in the educational mainstream.

In the past IEP documents and conferences did not resemble contemporary IEP practice, as the requirements have expanded over the years. As new legislation was passed, new mandates were added to the IEP process (see Chapter 7). And yet, despite all of the changes in legislation, which necessitate close collaboration between parents and schools, there is still often insufficient training to help teachers conduct effective conferences with parents. Furthermore, colleges and universities in the 1970s, 1980s, and even now fail to integrate relevant content into their programs to help teachers understand some of the unique demands placed on the family of a child with a disability. The purpose of this book is to contribute to the understanding and expertise of teachers and other school professionals involved in educating children with special needs.

The education of children with special needs has been revolutionized by the concept of inclusion—a philosophy that has led to greatly improved education for children. Early intervention programs and the implementation of IEPs have contributed to enriched and improved lives for children with disabilities. From a societal perspective, inclusion promises to reverse extant prejudice, exclusion, and stigma by creating a social environment for children that encourages healthy values toward "difference." Furthermore, I believe that it will promote social equality among future generations of children and adults who will grow into adolescence and adulthood without the burden of prejudice and with an ability to embrace difference.

Conducting Effective Conferences with Parents of Children with Disabilities is about two groups of people who must work together, often in the face of adversity—parents and teachers. The book is intended to help teachers better understand the lives of parents who are coping with and adapting to the ever changing needs of their children. The reader will learn that, just like all parents, parents of children with disabilities are deeply concerned about their children's current and future welfare, especially in the realm of education. Furthermore, the reader will understand more about the anxiety some parents have about their children's schooling. For some parents, anxieties and fears may prompt them to not show up for parent–teacher meetings or to arrive at conferences feeling defensive, confused, sad, or angry. Understanding these dynamics is essential for teachers in their quest to lead productive conferences with parents. The ultimate beneficiaries of effective collaboration between parents and teachers are the children whom both teachers and parents are striving to help.

Another major goal of the book is to provide teachers with

conferencing and interviewing tools to assist them in their quest to have productive meetings with parents. Just like parents, teachers may come to conferences with their own set of anxieties: How do I start a conference? How do I facilitate rapport with parents? What can I do to reduce my own anxiety? How do I handle differences of opinion? How can I cope with a "difficult" parent? Armed with useful strategies and ways of thinking about parents and families, teachers will be in a better position to promote empathy and rapport during conferences and feel more competent and at ease.

Perhaps the most productive way to use this book is to read the chapters sequentially. It is organized in a developmental fashion so that each chapter prepares the reader for the next one. Chapters 1 and 2 examine the relationship between families and schools over the years. These chapters establish a rationale for the implementation and merit of parent–teacher conferences. Chapter 2 also discusses how parents and teachers perceive each other, with a particular emphasis on how these reciprocal perceptions facilitate or detract from conferences.

In my view it is a futile task to understand families of children with disabilities without first studying fundamental family dynamic concepts, discussed in Chapter 3. A basic comprehension of family dynamics provides a solid foundation for grasping more complex family issues. The discussion of family dynamics is followed by Chapter 4, which explores family-related issues and dynamics specific to childhood disability and the family's response to it. Chapters 3 and 4 then form the foundation for understanding families by exploring such issues as the family life cycle, general coping mechanisms, family functions, and family structures. They also provide information on the mourning stages parents often experience when they first learn of their child's disabilities, the stresses associated with childhood disabilities, developmental transitions, and specific challenges to parents, siblings, and the extended family.

Chapter 5 establishes basic principles of interviewing, such as goal setting, facilitating rapport, consideration of the conference setting, and barriers to effective conferencing. Along the same lines, Chapter 6 illustrates more specific strategies, such as paraphrasing, timing issues, the effective use of questions, and understanding nonverbal responses during conferences. Chapter 7 explores the IEP process, which forms the fundamental content of most parent–teacher conferences. The rationale for IEP meetings is addressed, as well as the basic requirements outlined in recent changes in the law.

Chapter 8 explores characteristics of parents that may present challenges for teachers during conferences. Teachers may be anxious when conferring with angry or uncooperative parents. This chapter should help ease such concerns by examining ways to approach such parents. This chapter also explores some ethical concerns teachers may face during conferences and examines the issue of teacher burnout, an important topic considering the increasing demands and responsibilities teachers face. Preparing for and conducting parent conferences can be a daunting task.

Given the propensity of my wife, Karen, for detail and accuracy, and her special interest in disability issues, I enlisted her expertise in preparing the appendix, which lists disability-related agencies and books for children and parents. These resources represent a segment of the social support network surrounding families—resources that often are not known to family members—and can assist teachers in helping parents.

I am indebted to the secretaries who have worked on various chapters and versions of the manuscript for this book. My thanks go to Roberta Allen, Kim Morran, Mary Beth Merenick, and Cathy Trimbur. Their willingness to help when deadlines approached is greatly appreciated.

I owe much to my professional colleagues Fran Prezant, MEd, Charles Cohen, PhD, and Kaye Cupples, PhD, for their generosity in reading portions of the manuscript and providing helpful feedback. I am especially grateful for their assistance with Chapter 7. And, finally, I want to thank those with whom I worked at The Guilford Press—my editor, Chris Jennison, for keeping me on track; the copy editor, Jacquelyn Coggin, who contributed to the manuscript's readability; and the production editor, Anna Nelson, for her gentle guidance through the production process.

This book was written for the ultimate benefit of children with disabilities, their families, and the teachers and school professionals who work with these children. The central social context for improved lives for children is the family and, to a lesser yet crucial extent, the schools and the teachers who educate them.

Contents

Conducting Effective Conferences
with Parents of Children with Disabilities

1

Families and the Schools

There are numerous books and other resources to help teachers educate children. In recent years, the field of education has sought to broaden the context within which children acquire knowledge and personal growth by suggesting that teachers and other school personnel actively seek the cooperation of parents to extend and enrich children's learning experiences (Lambie & Daniels-Mohring, 1993; Fine & Carlson, 1992). There is little question that educators are supporting the active involvement of parents in both regular and special education (Reynolds & Birch, 1977; Losen & Diament, 1978; Rutherford & Edgar, 1979; Lombana, 1983; Simpson, 1996; Shea & Bauer, 1991). Actually, parental involvement in a child's education is not a new phenomenon. Its history goes back many centuries (Berger, 1981), but its importance is reemerging as an essential ingredient in child development.

Even though there is considerable sentiment that parental involvement is important and, in some instances, essential, only a modest effort is being directed toward how the school professional might engage parents in collaborative efforts. In both academic and applied settings, teachers are acquiring essential teaching skills but little, if any, training in working cooperatively with parents. One study surveyed 575 educators of teachers and found that only 4% taught a complete course on conferencing with parents, 15% reported offering part of a course on parents, and 37% reported having only one class on parent involvement (Chaukin & Williams, 1988).

In 1975, Kroth observed:

> Unfortunately, many teacher training programs do not provide an opportunity to students to learn the skills and techniques of conferring with parents. The importance of effective teacher/parent relationships cannot be overemphasized. Teachers who understand the children in their environment can make appropriate educational plans in the classroom. Parents who are provided with information about the school setting and their child's progress can be strong supporters and assistants in the child's educational growth and development. Parents and teachers who recognize each other's capabilities can join together in successful problem solving. (p. 155)

Others also agree that the development of effective school–family relationship skills is one component often missing from teacher training programs (Kaplan, 1992). In particular, students are rarely exposed to practical techniques to enhance these relationships (Rutherford & Edgar, 1979) even though there are now numerous resources that help professionals develop appropriate interpersonal skills (e.g., Nichols, 1995; Benjamin, 1987; Egan, 1998; Sommers-Flanagan & Sommers-Flanagan, 1993).

A decade after his 1975 book, Kroth (1985) noted in a publication that the home–school relationship continues to be problematic and in his view continues to be characterized by anger and mistrust:

> In many schools contacts with parents have decreased to the point where computer printouts of grades and an open house conducted early in the year represent the major communication between school and home. Concurrently, parent groups have been less supportive of educational systems. Bond issues have failed; adults in the communities have become more critical of pupil performance as measured by standardized tests; public school coaches have been relieved of their coaching duties for not producing winning teams; and educators have been taken to court for their placement procedures. (p. 1)

In this observation, Kroth argues that relations between the school and the family have become increasingly strained, making it even more incumbent for school professionals and parents to discover creative ways to work together on behalf of the children. But this will not be an easy task in this day and age, as social forces have created cross-currents of anger and mistrust. In the third edition, Kroth and Edge (1997) still lament the fact that parents continue to be outsiders in their child's education: "Parents continually have rated the educational systems below average and have cried out to be more involved in the daily lives of their children, but to no avail" (p. 1). Lombana (1983) agrees with Kroth's despairing view of home–school relationships by observing that

> the two institutions that most influence the growth and development of young people—the home and the school—are generally at odds with each other. At best, parents and school personnel conduct an uneasy and superficial alliance. Outward signs of cooperation and collaboration such as PTA, parents' councils, or similar organizations are too frequently mere appeasements designed to prevent open warfare. At its worst, open warfare *does* exist, represented by massive defeats of proposed school tax increases, public calls for the elimination of tenure for teachers, demands for administrator accountability, and a mass exodus of teachers from the classroom. More often, however, the situation is characterized by avoidance. Parents avoid educators because they don't understand them, feel threatened by them, and/or because they have little respect for them. Not surprisingly, school personnel behave the same way toward parents for the same reasons. (p. 2; emphasis added)

According to Kroth and Lombana, home–school relations, which are currently worsening, were never particularly amicable. In the past, these relationships were characterized by "creative conflict" rather than the "negative dissonance" so prevalent today (Lightfoot, 1981). Nevertheless, "teachers . . . who do not use parents as at least one-third of the learning team are utilizing only two-thirds of their potential effectiveness" (Buscaglia, 1975, p. 298). Simpson (1996) cites numerous studies suggesting that instructional programs are most effective when families and schools are supportive of each other and are able to build and maintain satisfactory lines of communication. Bradley, King-Sears, and Tessier-Switlick (1997) add that "parents are valuable sources of information, sometimes offering a broader perspective about students' strengths and needs in nonschool settings, strategies for dealing with behavioral challenges, key persons who may serve as resources, or ongoing stressors that may affect students' performance at school" (p. 330). And as Feldman, Byalick, and Rosedale (1975) add, "It is imperative that something be done to alter the negative conditions that have traditionally been present when parents and school officials are together" (p. 551). Adding to this observation, Rutherford and Edgar (1979) believe that the mistrust and hostility that characterize some parent–teacher relationships are due to three reasons:

1. The parents' fear of meeting the teacher. The reasons for this range from the parents' own negative school experiences, previous negative experiences with their child's teacher, and anxieties related to learning that their child is performing poorly and they are being blamed for the problems.
2. The media's persistent attack on the public schools.
3. The teachers' long-held belief that parents are responsible for the children's problems.

Naseef (1997) believes that conflict between parents and educators is common. He asserts that teachers' criticism of parents is also common because of their frustrations with students who have learning and behavior problems. After all, teachers are rewarded by children's successes and become frustrated and unsure of their competence when children do not learn efficiently, or when they manifest behavior problems. Naseef asserts that these failures that educators experience contribute to tense parent–teacher conferences. Hornby (1995) adds that teachers hold negative attitudes toward parents of children with disabilities because they view parents as problems and adversaries. Teachers see parents as less able, more vulnerable, and in need of treatment, and as causing or contributing to the child's disability. One mother observes that parents have a responsibility to enter into collaborative relationships with teachers—a collaboration that ultimately benefits their children:

> What I discovered was, no matter how skilled a teacher, how intuitive a therapist, how caring a principal, no one can know, nor have as much stake in the unique entity that is our child, as we as parents can. Therefore, we must enter into a partnership with the school system, become familiar with the terminology and knowledgeable about our rights and responsibilities. Having entered into this partnership, I feel confident, caring, effective, responsible, resourceful, and certainly more courageous. It's not always easy, but it is always necessary. Education is a process and we are all involved, whether we want to be or not. We will make mistakes along the way, but we cannot remain bystanders. (Bradley et al., 1997, p. 102)

Parents who remain "bystanders" or are not actively involved in their children's education jeopardize their children's futures. However, as I mention later, not all parents have the personal or environmental resources to become involved in their child's education. In this regard, Bradley et al. (1997) state, "When a parent makes the decision to have minimal involvement, the [school] team must respect that right. When a parent decides to become highly involved, teams can capitalize on that participation rather than become threatened by it" (p. 105). These authors alert teachers to expect conflict, but to try to remain nonjudgmental and respectful. They offer the following suggestions that have proven helpful in conducting parent conferences and team meetings that include parents, teachers, and other involved school personnel:

- Expect conflict to arise.
- Deal with conflict through consensus building.
- Respect and solicit parent input frequently in meetings.
- Expect that you won't have all the answers.
- Begin meetings with ideas—not a completed plan.
- Avoid jargon.
- Communicate frequently with parents and keep many of the communications positive.
- Be patient—parents may have trouble getting their ideas across to the team, and they may be tense or angry.
- Keep meeting times flexible.
- Use round robin style sharing during the meeting.
- Assist parents with concerns at home whenever possible. (p. 105)

In working with parents, a major concern is the tendency to increase the roles and functions assumed by teachers and other school personnel, thereby overburdening them. They are expected to share many of the responsibilities previously assigned exclusively to parents. This trend may reflect a discomfort with perceived gaps in adequate parenting or suggest that the parenting that takes place in the home should be reinforced in school. Some researchers believe that due to the numerous roles and responsibilities that parents assume, they must depend on others outside the family to help with parenting (Shea & Bauer, 1991). Others believe that teachers should serve as allies in the parents' efforts to raise their children. In this regard, Berger (1981) cites several large-scale studies that show that rather than school curricula and expenditures on facilities and materials, it is the quality of the teaching and the parents' support of education that affect school achievement. Moreover, parent education and involvement seem to have a salutary effect on the cognitive, affective, and social development of children (Bronfenbrenner, 1979). According to Harry (1992), many studies have concluded that family environments are more influential in children's school progress than the schools. Because the family is so significant to a child's learning endeavors, school professionals should make every effort to collaborate with parents, so that the most influential factor in a child's schooling, namely, the parents, is not alienated.

The fact is that whether school professionals wish to or not, they are required by law (Public Laws 94-142 and 99-457) to confer with parents about the special needs of their children. Public Law 94-142, passed in 1975, relates directly to parents and the schools, as teachers are periodically required to review with parents the child's Individualized Education Program (IEP). Public Law 99-457 focuses more on the family unit, as professionals employed in early intervention programs must conduct a family needs assessment to help design appropriate treatment strategies (Marion, 1992; Seligman & Darling, 1997). Essentially, Public Law 99-457 extended the rights and privileges of Public Law 94-142 downward. The net effect of these major pieces of legislation has been to bring the family and the school together in a coequal partnership from the birth of the child through 21 years of his or her life. Thus, while the rift between families and schools seems to be intensifying, major legislative initiatives are requiring these two entities to work together in the interests of the children (Simpson & Kamps, 1996).

INCLUSION

Another key reason to work cooperatively with parents is related to the concept of inclusion. The inclusion movement, which has been subject to debate (Bradley et al., 1997), asserts that children with a wide variety of disabilities be included in regular classrooms. This has implications for regular education teachers and their preparedness to work with these children *and their parents*.

Attitudinal studies in the 1980s showed that educators support a more segregated model than what supporters of inclusion endorse. In more recent studies, the perceptions of elementary and secondary general and special education teachers and administrators with experience in inclusion-oriented schools favored the education of children with disabilities in general education. They supported this position in the context of a shared, collaborative relationship between general and special education. It is important to note that teacher support came *after* they achieved the expertise needed to implement this initiative. No matter what the data from the studies show, it is clear that the inclusion model is and will continue to be the subject of continuing debate. Simpson (1996) offers a set of guidelines that educators and parents may wish to bear in mind as they consider inclusion for a child. The interested reader may wish to consult Simpson on this topic, as it is beyond the scope of this book to discuss the numerous issues involved in inclusion.

It seems crucial to the success of an integrative model of education that educators be prepared. And part of that preparation involves training both regular and special education teachers in the principles of effective conferencing skills. It is also imperative that teachers be informed about the common and unique features of these families' dynamics, especially those that exist when there is a child with a disability residing in the home.

WHAT IS THE TEACHER'S ROLE?

With these forces impinging on teachers today, a teacher may ask, "Am I supposed to be a teacher of children, a surrogate parent, a 'counselor' to parents, or all of these?" The response would probably be "all of these," with the qualification that teachers should be considered facilitators in parent–teacher conferences and not "counselors" who provide psychological services. Furthermore, the training of teachers as competent conference leaders and facilitators to parents must be an integral part of any training program for prospective teachers. This notion runs concurrent with the push to have pediatricians, who, of course, have already mastered their craft from a medical point of view, become more knowledgeable about and comfortable with the family members of chronically ill or disabled children they treat. They are often in a position of communicating to family members upsetting information that has lifelong implications.

No matter how resistant teachers, other staff, and parents may be to parent conferences, sooner or later, the school will be faced with parents who carry the responsibility of the day-to-day care and development of their child with a disability. Since parent–teacher conferences are inevitable, and because it would be most desirable to have them and conduct them in an effective manner, it is to the school's advantage to support them actively and to be adequately prepared to conduct them. This volume, then, is an effort to help staff in educational institutions deal as effectively with parents of children they teach as they do with the children they instruct.

A FAMILY SYSTEMS PERSPECTIVE

The field of family therapy has long embraced family systems thinking in efforts to help families understand and cope with problems they face. A disruptive child is not seen as the client in therapy. Instead, the family unit is seen as the client and efforts are made to include family members in treatment, not just the child. Related to educational institutions, the family systems view encourages schools to have a greater awareness of the power of the family in creating, maintaining, or lessening school-related problems. Furthermore, a systems perspective asserts that there are interdependent, interacting systems that can fuel or help to alleviate child problems if the family and school cooperate ultimately to benefit the child. Accordingly, a problem is best understood when seen as an adaptation of the child's relationships within the family, and relatedly, as the child's ability to cope with the vicissitudes of the family–school relationship (Fine & Carlson, 1992). This, then, makes it imperative that educational institutions and families view each other as allies rather than as adversaries.

To look at the school–home connection another way, when dysfunctional behavior is practiced within the family, related settings such as the schools and, reciprocally, from schools to the family, are affected. "In short from the systems perspective, the etiology and maintenance of the school—related problematic behavior is not considered to be child based but rather is considered to be based contextually in the immediate and extended sets of relationships in which the child is embedded. Thus, systems practitioners frequently involve families in school-based problems and involve schools in family-based problems" (Fine & Carlson, 1992, p. xi).

THE RESPONSIBILITY
FOR PARENT–TEACHER CONFERENCES

A particularly important focus in parent–teacher meetings is on the cooperative *educational* venture, that is, parents and teachers and other school personnel working together on a child's educational program. In this regard, Reynolds and Birch (1977) reiterate the value of good school–family relationships by noting that "there is increasing evidence that a child's educational progress is accelerated when teachers and parents work in close partnership" (p. 175). Their view supporting positive school–family relationships is now echoed in numerous publications (Lambie & Daniels-Mohring, 1993; Hornby, 1995; Shea & Bauer, 1991; Alper, Schloss, & Schloss, 1994; Harry, 1992; Simpson, 1996).

During a conference, the focus is generally on the educational program that is carried out in the home. The teacher may wish to schedule a conference with parents to discuss the child's progress and how family members can help the child at home, or to communicate specific concerns related to the child's behavior, attendance, how best to approach a learning task, and so forth. Conversely, on their own initiative, parents may ask for a meeting to discuss the child's schoolwork; to inform the teacher of changes in their child's progress or changes perceived in their child's behavior at home; to gain support, encouragement, or information; or because they are upset or angry at the school. Other professionals in the school (e.g., social worker, psychologist, or counselor) may recommend that a meeting be held with the social worker, parents, and teacher present.

Meetings, then, may be initiated by a number of different involved persons for a variety of reasons, but the responsibility for the liaison between parents and the school rests squarely on the shoulders of the teacher: "Communicating with and guiding parents is now an integral part of the teacher's responsibility. Other school staff members (counselors, social workers, principals, psychologists, supervisors) may assume some of the responsibility, but in the final analysis it is the teacher–parent interaction that is essential" (Reynolds & Birch, 1977, p. 183).

GIVING SUPPORT AND ENCOURAGEMENT

Teachers may be confronted with dispirited parents experiencing considerable doubt, confusion, and anxiety about their child with a disability and their reactions to her. A troubled parent may enlist the help of a teacher to discuss problems that are related to a child's performance at school or other, more personal concerns that bear a relationship to the child. A parent's inability to cope effectively with a child is often a motivating factor in seeking help. A person may feel embarrassed to engage a psychologist or other mental health specialist, or be unable to afford one. Other services may not be known to parents, or they may feel that with regard to their child, the teacher is the most knowledgeable professional; thus, the teacher may find the distraught parent at her doorstep.

A teacher's initial reaction to meeting with parents might justifiably be one of anxiety. For most teachers, this anxiety is rooted in the partially realistic fear that they may not be able to cope with the situation because they feel ill-prepared to cope with a parent meeting.

When parents are obviously distressed, the strategy of actively listening and being supportive and encouraging may be (and often is) all that is necessary. When someone is troubled, often the best strategy is to be an attentive, understanding, nonjudgmental listener (Nichols, 1995). Of course, when it is obvious that some sort of intervention beyond the teacher's expertise is needed, the teacher's support should be augmented by concrete suggestions as to where assistance may be sought. The suggestion for counseling, for example, should be accompanied by an explanation of why counseling can be helpful. For example, a professional might say, "It seems that taking care of David is a 24-hour a day job. What makes it worse is that your husband has been despondent over his mother's death and hasn't been able to help with David as much as he has in the past. You told me that he has been depressed for 3 months now. I wonder if you've considered counseling to help you and your husband cope with this situation." Although a teacher who suggests counseling may encounter some resistance, this resistance should be substantially diminished when the referral is made by a competent, caring, and understanding teacher. And, indeed, such a recommendation may be a welcome anchor in stressful times.

EFFECT OF TEACHERS

In the field of counseling/psychotherapy, it was generally thought that counselors or psychologists had either a positive influence on their clients or none whatsoever. Eysenck's (1955) landmark rebuttal to a number of research studies he examined on psychotherapy outcomes revealed that people improved or remained essentially the same regardless of psychotherapeutic intervention. The assertion that psychotherapy had little effect on people shocked the professional community, but the point to be made here is that no mention was made of the possible deleterious effect therapy might have had on some clients.

In a later examination of the same studies that Eysenck reviewed,

Bergin (1963) discovered that although some people did indeed improve and others did not change, a number of the treated group actually *declined in their social–emotional adjustment.* This was the first empirically based conclusion that clients under psychotherapeutic treatment might improve, remain essentially unchanged, or get worse. Later, after a number of studies, Carkhuff (1969) concluded that as a consequence of therapeutic treatment, client outcomes might be "for better or for worse." The idea is frightening that people are harmed in a situation theoretically designed to bring about growth. These revelations, along with reports that some participants in small psychotherapeutic groups found themselves less well off after than before the experience (Yalom, 1995; Yalom & Lieberman, 1971), have made the profession of psychology examine more carefully the variables that account for effective therapeutic change.

Although the effectiveness of counseling and psychotherapy is no longer unquestioned, Eysenck's criticism has served the profession positively. Practicing clinicians and graduate training programs have responded by evaluating counseling outcomes more diligently and explaining the process by which they are achieved. By the way, after over 40 years of evaluating counseling and psychotherapy outcomes, it is clear that most clients do indeed benefit from the experience (Whiston & Sexton, 1993, "Does Therapy Help," 1995). Furthermore, we now know that the therapeutic *relationship,* is critical to positive client outcome. This compelling fact has clear relevance to educators who confer with parents.

What implications do these observations have for teachers? For one thing, the question of teacher effectiveness has to be addressed in a much more serious fashion than in the past. The possibility that teachers, like counselors, may have a negative effect (recall Bergin's contention that some people in counseling actually get worse) on children must be examined, and careful attention must be given to certain characteristics or behaviors that bear a relationship to effective or ineffective teaching. Also, if it is possible for teachers to have a negative impact on children, they may also have the same effect on parents during conferences.

A study some time ago by Branan (1972) presented some compelling evidence that teachers must be aware of the relationships they establish with their pupils in the classroom. Branan asked 150 college-age students to describe in detail what they considered the two most negative experiences in their lives. Negative experiences were considered to be those that the respondents felt made their lives worse or were a negative force in their development. Responses were divided into two categories: interpersonal and nonpersonal experiences. Out of 300 responses, 257 involved interpersonal relationships, and the largest subcategory was interaction with teachers. Recentness of experience was not an important variable; more negative experiences occurred in high school than in college, and in elementary than in junior high school. Teachers were involved more often than any other persons in the most negative experiences reported, with parents a poor second. Individual situations included humiliation in front of the class, unfairness in evaluation, destruction of self-confidence, personality conflicts, and embarrassment. Branan concluded that "human relations training and skill should be as important a prerequisite for teachers as any other requirement. Human relations knowledge and skill should become a prerequisite to teacher credentials at any level. The damage resulting from sarcastic, insensitive, and noncaring teachers at any level must be decreased" (p. 82).

Harmful learning environments probably occur most often in instances of difference in race, social class, and disability. In her book *Cultural Diversity, Families, and the Special Education System*, with data from numerous studies, Beth Harry (1992) documents that children who vary from the norm are often taught in unhealthy classroom settings. In the conclusion to her book, Harry writes:

> This study can only recommend that the field move toward services based on descriptions of students' needs rather than on the ascribing of disability classifications that stigmatize children. Ethnic minority students already have the burden of battling stigmatizing labels as they struggle to move out of their position at the bottom of the social and economic ladder of the United States. The literature increasingly shows that cultural differences are devalued by an educational system bent on identifying deficits rather than strengths and that the insistence on identifying a rigid border between normality and disability is at best erroneous, at worst malicious. (p. 246)

Although it is obviously important for a teacher to be skilled in the methods of instruction, in the past there was an overemphasis on instructional methods and an underemphasis on the development of proper learning climates related to learning and achievement. There has been an increase in publications addressed to the social and psychological impact teachers have on their charges. Nonetheless, university curricula continue to emphasize teaching methodology, while facilitative interpersonal skills are largely ignored.

It is essential in teaching and in conducting parent–teacher conferences that teachers pay more attention to relationship issues. Most teachers apparently know and can talk about the importance of being a helping person, but few are capable of putting theory into practice without training. Based on a number of published studies, Combs, Blume, Newman, and Wass (1974) concluded that good teachers share the following characteristics:

1. perceive others as having the capacity to deal with their problems successfully.
2. do not regard others as threatening [to themselves] but rather [see them] as essentially well-intentioned.
3. see other people as being worthy rather than unworthy.
4. see people as creative and dynamic rather than passive or inert.
5. regard [people's] behavior as understandable rather than capricious, unpredictable, or negative.
6. regard people as important sources of satisfaction rather than sources of frustration and suspicion. (p. 63)

Over a period of 4 years, Wittmer and Myrick (1974) collected open-ended responses from undergraduate and graduate college students regarding their experiences with teachers, from which the authors were able to extract lists of adjectives (p. 39) that characterized good and poor teachers. According to the students, ineffective teachers had the following qualities:

1. Insensitive
2. Cold
3. Disinterested
4. Authoritarian
5. Ridiculing
6. Arbitrary
7. Sarcastic
8. Demanding
9. Punitive
10. Disciplinarian

The effective teachers had the following qualities:

1. Good listeners
2. Empathetic
3. Caring
4. Concerned
5. Genuine

6. Warm
7. Interested
8. Knowledgeable
9. Trusting
10. Friendly
11. Sense of humor
12. Dynamic
13. Able to communicate

Aspy and Roebuck (1967) spent a number of years studying the effect teachers have on their students. Aspy was particularly intrigued with Carl Rogers's conception of the ingredients required to successfully conduct individual psychotherapy. Rogers believed that if the psychotherapist could communicate high levels of empathy, congruence, and positive regard, constructive changes would follow. Rogers, by the way, was one of the first prominent theoreticians to put his theory to empirical test. The dimensions of empathy (E), congruence (C), and positive regard (PR) were operationally defined by Rogers, who then proceeded to develop ways to measure them.

Empathy is defined as one's ability to perceive and recognize the inner feelings and experiences of another. It has been characterized as "walking in another person's shoes." In addition to sensing a person's feelings, empathy includes the ability to respond to someone else so as to communicate that the nature and intensity of an emotion is understood.

Congruence refers to the consistency between one's beliefs, attitudes, feelings, and values, and one's behavior. For example, an illustration of incongruence would be a teacher saying, "I really love working with the parents of the children I teach," yet experiencing considerable apprehension before and during parent conferences.

Positive regard refers to accepting another person unconditionally no matter what his attributes or values happen to be. For example, a teacher is as accepting of a parent who dresses, talks, and has a belief system different from hers as she would be of a parent who more closely resembles her. In this regard, Simpson (1990) observed, "Professionals will come into contact with children, parents and families who represent a variety of value systems, some of which may be dramatically different from their own. Recognition of this possibility is critical if the educational conference is to work effectively with children, parents, and families with variant socioeconomic, religious, ethnic, cultural, and political persuasions" (p. 14).

Because teaching, like counseling, includes building rapport, Aspy was persuaded to use these three constructs to determine the effect low and high E, C, and PR teachers have on their students.

One study investigated the relationship between the teacher's level of facilitative interpersonal conditions (E, C, PR) and the cognitive growth of third-grade students (Aspy, 1969). The results indicated that teachers who provide high levels of facilitative conditions tend to increase students' cognitive growth, but those who provide low levels of these conditions tend to retard learning. A replication of the study confirmed the findings. The data also revealed that low-functioning teachers reported significantly more student absences than high-functioning ones, which led the authors to speculate that there may be some relationship between school phobia and the interpersonal skills of the teacher.

Another study indicated that students' use of their higher cognitive processes (e.g., problem solving) is significantly and positively related to the teacher's levels of interpersonal conditions (Aspy & Roebuck, 1967). This relationship was particularly strong for positive regard, prompting the authors to speculate that since thinking aloud is a kind of interpersonal risk, persons tend to do it more frequently when they feel valued.

Additional studies by Aspy and others (Ivey, 1983; Egan, 1990, 1998) indicate that for teachers to improve their interpersonal skills they must have supervisors and professors who rate high in these skills themselves. Educators whose level of skills is low have a deleterious effect on those they train, just as teachers who have poor facilitative skills have a negative impact on their pupils. It bears repeating that this conclusion appears to be as true in teaching as it is in counseling.

Just like in counseling/psychotherapy, one might hypothesize that teacher–parent relationships may likewise be either positive or negative. Given the fact that teachers receive little formal training in interpersonal processes, and aside from teachers who are naturally gifted communicators, there is a chance that some teachers are relatively ineffective in dealing with parents. Teachers who work with parents of children with disabilities, in particular, often are confronted by difficult and complex situations. Hence, the need to develop good interpersonal skills is apparent. Carl Rogers, as quoted by Lyon (1971), makes this point most poignantly: "Better courses, better curricula, better coverage, better teaching machines will never resolve our dilemma in a basic way. Only persons acting like persons in their relationships with their students (and parents) can even begin to make a dent on this most urgent problem of modern education" (p. 251).

ADMINISTRATORS AND THE
HOME–SCHOOL RELATIONSHIP

Perhaps the most potent source of support for teachers is principals and other administrative personnel responsible for the management of a school. The point of view (philosophy or theoretical orientation) of the administration trickles down through the hierarchy to staff and faculty employees. Powerful norms* in a school setting, or any organization for that matter, which reflect the conscious or unconscious desires of the managers of the organization, have an impact on the philosophy and practices of a school.

For the sake of the children, parents, and teachers in an educational institution, one would hope that administrative support exists for cordial and helpful relationships between the school and home. It is important for administrators to sanction and indeed encourage teachers to work collaboratively and facilitatively with parents. Such an attitude (or norm) will do much to further the teacher's feeling that what she is doing is condoned by the school and reinforce the idea that good parent–teacher relationships are beneficial and have broad support. In this regard, Lyon (1971) observes that "if our schools and our educational systems are managed by less than human managers, we cannot expect our teachers to be humanistic in their orientation. Accordingly, emphasis on people-oriented management must begin at the top echelons and flow down if it is to have any positive effect on teachers" (p. 251).

In terms of inclusion practices, Bradley et al. (1997) argue that "a crucial factor is gaining administrative support. Superintendents as well as building principals must understand, support, and be able to explain the reasons for establishing inclusive schools" (p. 10). Thus, for any major thrust in education, it is imperative that administrators be well informed and genuinely supportive of the effort. Others concur that administrative blessings help to ensure the implementation of programs (Lambie & Daniels-Mohring, 1993).

Berger (1981) believes that administrative leadership is manifested

---

*"Norms are the rules of behavior, the proper ways of acting in a group that have been accepted as legitimate by the members of the group" (Napier & Gershenfeld, 1981, p. 122).

in four aspects of school–parent collaboration. He says that the esprit de corps of the school and staff reflect the administrator's ability to build morale. It is the administrators task to help staff members feel positive and enthusiastic about working with children and secure in their work with both children and their parents. The second role, program designer, involves the implementation of the educational program. The administrator needs to encourage home–school relationships as an integral part of the educational program. The third role has to do with the administrator's ability to make the parent feel welcome at school by subscribing to an open-door policy, scheduling open houses, arranging for parent education meetings, and the like. In the fourth role the administrator is a program coordinator to ensure that parent involvement programs continue to be valued and implemented.

Shea and Bauer (1991) believe that administrative support is essential:

> School administrators and special education directors and supervisors can provide considerable logistical support by granting official permission to start a parent program, setting aside time for the program, supplying facilities, equipment, materials, and so on. They may help draw in parents as well as school and community consultants to the program and offer social and emotional support through public recognition of efforts. (p. 103)

In terms of collaboration between regular and special education teachers, Reeve and Hallahan (1996, cited in Meyan, Vergason, & Whelan, 1996, p. 412) assert that "the need for administrative support for collaborative arrangements between general and special educators is proclaimed repeatedly in the literature. Administrative leadership sets the tone for innovative practices and their acceptance by teachers who follow the administrative lead."

SCHOOL CLIMATE AND SCHOOL ADMINISTRATORS

Some cues that reveal whether a particular school projects a facilitative climate include the following:

1. Is the school a positive and exciting place to learn and to be with others?

2. Do the children make positive or negative comments about the
   school, the teacher, the principal, and themselves?
3. Do teachers and administration discuss their school and the
   students in a positive fashion, or are there suggestions of a serious morale problem?
4. Does the rapport among and between teachers and school administrators seem poor or good?

In a study using the School Survey of Interpersonal Relationships
(SSIR) with 211 elementary and secondary schools in Florida, Wittmer
(1971) showed that a school's climate of learning is largely determined
by the relationship between (1) the teacher and the principal, (2) the
teacher and other teachers, (3) the teacher and other helping personnel,
and (4) the teacher and students.

The atmosphere of a school is largely dependent on the administration, and the central figure in promulgating a facilitative climate for
other administrators, staff, teachers, and students is the principal.

> A facilitative principal knows the need for close communication be-
> tween himself and the teachers. He knows that teachers need support
> and reassurance. He senses that there is a time to evaluate and a time
> to respond to feelings as well as ideas and products. He is eager to
> communicate with teachers in time of excitement and satisfaction, as
> well as in time of crisis. A facilitative principal has all of the character-
> istics of a facilitative teacher. (Wittmer & Myrick, 1974, p. 150)

Another writer singles out the principal for having a major impact
on a school's philosophy, stating unequivocally that "the principal is
the greatest determinant of the character of the school" (Blake, 1977, p.
120).

Perhaps the most important lesson to be learned from this discussion is that school administrators need to be committed to the value of
parent conferences and to make allowances for a diversity of ideas and
practices. "The choice . . . is not between whether to include parents or
to exclude them but whether to include them grudgingly or to develop
new strategies for working with parents to achieve important mutual
goals" (Losen & Diament, 1978, p. 4). An atmosphere where open communication is valued, and innovation and experimentation are encouraged, would be conducive to facilitative and positive relationships extending from administrators to teachers, to students, and, ultimately,
to parents. A positive atmosphere is particularly critical when teachers

are dealing with students who have special needs and parents, as a consequence of their child's needs, have added burdens that they sometimes bring to the teacher.

INFLUENCING A RELUCTANT SYSTEM

When the administration is inflexible and views parents as nuisances, teachers may wish to consider ways of persuading the administration and other faculty and staff that working productively with parents of children with disabilities is important. Faculty meetings would seem to be a particularly good place for a teacher to discuss parent conferences he has had. An astute teacher can indicate the connection between positive teacher–parent relationships and a child's academic, social, and emotional growth.

Social modeling is one of the best methods of influencing others who lack competence and self-confidence. Teachers who have experience communicating with parents can encourage other teachers who may be anxious about conferring with parents to observe them conducting parent–teacher conferences. After observing a good model for a number of conferences, the reluctant teacher can ask that same person, or someone else she admires and with whom she feels comfortable, for supervision as she takes on the responsibility herself. Another possibility would be to ask an outside consultant to help train or supervise staff in parent conferencing.

Tape recordings of sessions can be very helpful to staff members and allow others (teachers and administrators) to take part in parent conferences. This participation is easily accomplished by asking for suggestions or recommendations from colleagues after playing a recording (e.g., "How would you handle this kind of a situation?" or "Can anybody think of alternative ways I might have handled this situation?"). Admittedly, it would take a courageous person to risk this kind of feedback, but the effort could help dissipate resistance about conferring with parents.

In taping a conference, the teacher must be sure to ask the parent(s) if they would mind being taped and discuss with them how the tapes will be used. For example, a teacher could tell the parents that the sessions are being recorded so that he could replay the tape later for learning purposes with other teachers. He might also inform them that the school occasionally asks parent's permission to be recorded so that teachers can improve their conferencing skills. If others will be listening to the tape, the teacher must so inform the parents. Taping should never be done without some *training* goal in mind, and the confidentially of the parents must always be respected.

HUMAN CHARACTERISTICS AND DEVELOPMENT OF A PROFESSIONAL HELPER

A popular theory in vocational psychology is that people seek occupations that fulfill certain psychological needs. Individuals who enter the helping professions are no exception. Teachers, like counselors, are attracted to their field because it enables them to gratify their desire to be helpful, needed, and appreciated by others. In addition, the need to be seen as knowledgeable, likable, and as having a certain amount of status and influence may be present. On a darker note, the selection of a person-oriented profession by some individuals may be motivated by the need to know about the private lives of others from a position of authority, or the need to have clients or children make up for the emptiness that characterizes their personal or social lives.

Whatever the need, relatively few in the helping professions are "gifted" or "natural" helpers, communicators, or facilitators. Because of their upbringing, education, or the models present during the developmental years (e.g., parents, teachers, respected peers), a minority of the professionals who work with people have a naturally warm, understanding, and generally trusting manner. Such people, although they can profit by further sharpening their interpersonal skills, have little need for extensive training. On the other hand, because of the developmental influences mentioned earlier, most of us have to work conscientiously at functioning optimally during interpersonal endeavors such as conferencing. This need is particularly critical for teachers who must work effectively with their pupils, some of whom are disabled, *and* the parents of these children—a most demanding job.

In summary, three ingredients must be present to help teachers work effectively with children who have disabilities and their parents: (1) a thorough understanding of the dynamics of families who have a child with a disability; (2) a good cognitive understanding of the dimensions of effective interpersonal relationships, combined with opportunities to practice communication skills; and (3) extensive experience working with parents of children with disabilities.

A firm grasp of family dynamics combined with interpersonal skills development provide the teacher with the knowledge and skills needed for effective conferencing. No reading or training can take the place of the actual experience of working with parents. As experience accumulates (given a sound foundation), the teacher's effectiveness and feelings of ease will increase.

Before moving into an examination of family dynamics in Chapters 3 and 4, Chapter 2 explores prevailing attitudes teachers have toward parents. Particular emphasis is placed on reciprocal teacher–parent attitudes. To grasp the nature of such relationships, it is important to be aware of the needs and stresses of both parties. An analysis of what parents and teachers bring to their mutual relationship from historical, psychological, and sociological perspectives should help teachers begin to understand and cope with a situation that sometimes is fraught with considerable apprehension.

2

Parents and Teachers: Reciprocal Views

$\mathbf{A}$t the risk of oversimplification, one might surmise that human beings respond to each other out of a combination of reality factors and stereotypical beliefs. Examples of behavior that reflect objective phenomena (or reality) include overt hostile responses, such as a sharp exchange between two strangers at a football game or the fear shown by a snake-phobic person to the sight of a reptile. In contrast, responses indicative of attitudes based on stereotypes are represented by assigning certain attitudes and behaviors to specific ethnic and minority groups, to people of different socioeconomic levels, or to children and adolescents with disabilities.

Perceptions of certain situations tend to be fairly universal; that is, many people would perceive a physical assault as an expression of hostility; whereas stereotypes, although they may be held by groups of people, are reflections of more individualized or idiosyncratic reactions. Stereotypes are largely the product of interactions with significant others during one's formative years, and they may be reinforced by peer influences, political associations, religious affiliations, and the like (Marshak & Seligman, 1993).

In dealing with the schools, poor, minority parents of children with disabilities are at a triple disadvantage in that reality factors such as poverty intersect with prejudice toward persons with certain attributes (Harry, 1992). As Herman (1983) puts it, "When the three status distinctions of poverty, minority, and childhood exceptionality intersect, the families involved are uniquely vulnerable to systematic discrimination" (p. 47).

How teachers perceive students and how teachers and parents perceive each other are subject to a complex combination of factors. Because attitudes are the precursors to behavior, and because behavior often reveals underlying attitudes, it is instructive to study reciprocal attitudes held by school personnel and the populations they serve. In this discussion, particular attention is given to reciprocal parent–teacher attitudes and how such perceptions influence their relationship. However, this chapter begins with a brief examination of teacher attitudes toward students. These attitudes are the seeds from which beliefs about family members are born.

TEACHERS' ATTITUDES TOWARD PUPILS

An overview of this topic should serve a twofold purpose: to ascertain how the attitudes of classroom teachers facilitate or impede learning, and, perhaps more crucial to the focus of this book, to determine whether a relationship exists between teacher-held attitudes toward students and those held toward parents.

Stern and Keislar (1977) warn that the research in this area spans a wide range of sophistication; some studies reflect questionable reliability and often use inadequate instruments for gathering data. A starting point for this discussion is a quotation from Kaplan (1992), who notes that

> study after study indicates . . . that poor teaching is rarely attributable to poor content background. Incompetent teaching seems more to be a matter of poor organization, less than adequate management techniques, and *little concern for the affective needs of student*. More simply stated, some teachers are dull, unimaginative, and seemingly uninterested in the backgrounds, feelings, and needs of their students . . . In a world growing in complexity, it is no longer acceptable to prepare teachers the way it has always been done. Far more is required to meet the cognitive needs of our children with their other needs as learners. Business as usual will not suffice. (p. 230; emphasis added)

Although teachers' attitudes toward students are said to have an effect on how students feel about themselves as well as how they view their academic development, Khan and Weiss (1972), in their review of the literature, indicate that there is very little direct evidence to demonstrate this relationship. The conclusions of their review may be indicative of the difficulty in measuring teachers' attitudes and students' reactions to them. In contrast, and perhaps a reflection of 20 years of research since the Kahn and Weiss review, Harry (1992) asserts that a considerable body of literature supports the belief that racial bias is endemic to the behavior of many teachers. She cites studies of teachers' impressions of hypothetical cases that have shown that teachers expect special class placement more frequently for Mexican Americans than for Anglo students. Other studies of teacher–student interactions have demonstrated higher rates of teacher attention and praise to Anglo children and negative teacher attitudes toward non-English native speakers (Buriel, 1983; Jackson & Cosca, 1974).

The authors of a study of Hmong children in California report that a prejudicial school environment led to the isolation of ethnic children:

> Racial prejudice about the ability of Indochinese children, whether conscious or unconscious, is deeply rooted in the misperception by mainstream teachers and peers that these children are academically incompetent because they have an inferior intelligence or an inferior culture, not because they have a different set of experiences leading to different values and cognitive system. (Trueba, Jacobs, & Kirton, 1990, p. 103)

Different attitudes are elicited from teachers by certain attributes of students, the most important being race or ethnicity, socioeconomic status, divergent speech patterns or language, level of ability or achievement, sex, and classroom behavior (Stern & Keislar, 1977).

Related to race, there are reports indicating that both white and black teachers have biased attitudes toward black students (Swick & Lamb, 1972), and that their attitudes toward Mexican American students are also extremely negative (Harry, 1992). Black children are described as being more introverted, more distractible, and more hostile than white children, and Mexican American children are seen by teachers as possessing a negative self-concept (Palomares, 1970).

Students who present behavior problems are treated differently, depending upon whether they come from middle-class or poor families (Stern & Keislar 1977). Parent conferences are more generally the rule with students of higher socioeconomic status, whereas with the poor child, more emphasis is placed on punitive action.

Speech is often confounded with race and socioeconomic status, and it has particular relevance to teachers working with children with disabilities who have expressive disorders. The literature supports the finding that communication patterns affect teachers' perceptions of students (Cohen & Kimmerling, 1971). Furthermore, judgments based on speech characteristics tend to be predictive of how children are graded and assigned to classrooms (Williams, Whitehead, & Miller, 1971).

There are studies indicating that gender stereotyping is an important determinant of differential attitudes. Current emphasis on sexual equality may bring into question the extent to which previously reported attitudes are still extant. Nevertheless, the evidence indicates that teachers have negative attitudes and expectations toward boys even before they enter the classroom, and that boys receive more disapproval than girls (Zach & Price, 1973). For the most part, however, students, whatever their sex, who are considered conforming, obedient, compliant, quiet, studious, and passive are generally preferred by teachers (Stern & Keislar, 1977).

In a study sponsored by the U.S. Commission on Civil Rights (1974, cited in Smith, 1979), the classroom interactions of teachers with Mexican American and Anglo American children were observed in nearly 500 classrooms in the Southwestern United States. The results of this study showed the following:

1. Teachers praised Anglo-Americans 36 percent more often than they praised Mexican-Americans;
2. Teachers used or built upon the ideas of Anglo-American students 40 percent more frequently than they used or built upon the ideas of Mexican-American students;
3. Teachers responded 40 percent more positively to Anglo-American than to Mexican-American students;
4. Teachers directed questions to Anglo-Americans 21 percent more often than to Mexican-Americans;
5. Teachers spent 23 percent more time in all in non-disapproving talk with Anglo-American than with Mexican-American students;
6. The average Anglo-American spent approximately 27 percent more time speaking in the classroom than did the average Mexican-American student. (Smith, 1979, pp. 40–41)

With children from low-socioeconomic-status or minority back-grounds, teacher communications tend to focus on controlling/man-aging classroom behavior, while with majority, middle-class children, teacher communications are more relevant to the content or skills of in-struction (Harry, 1992; Henderson, 1980; Laosa, 1977). In this regard, research has shown that student achievement is related to the nature of teacher–student interactions (Hoge & Luce, 1979). An illustration of this is the significant drop in achievement levels of high-achieving Mexican American students when they had teachers identified as high in discrimination (Johnson, Gerard, & Miller, 1975).

As Stern and Keislar indicate, the attitude of the teacher has been identified in many studies as the critical variable in student learning and development. Attitudes formed by cultural factors, socioeconomic status, sex, and ability constitute an important consideration in teach-ing children with exceptionalities (Harry, 1992; Lynch & Lewis, 1988). Attitudes that lead to negative expectations are compounded by atti-tudes generated by deviations from the norm, such as disfigurement, different speaking and walking patterns, and expression of realistic dependency by some students with disabilities and those whose learn-ing is impeded (Marshak & Seligman, 1993). To complicate the situa-tion, these attitudinal predispositions have little chance for change be-cause of existing pressures on the teacher, such as unfavorable class size, disciplinary problems, and inadequate preparation to deal with the wide range of students teachers are required to educate. The prob-lems for teachers are formidable, as they are being asked to take on more responsibility, assume added roles, and learn new skills.

In conclusion, it is possible to say with considerable certainty that negative attitudes exist toward students with certain characteristics. These attitudes affect children academically and psychologically. Atti-tudes are often subtly expressed: therefore, their impact is difficult to as-certain in empirical studies. Nevertheless, negative attitudes of teachers toward children do little to enhance children's confidence and self-esteem or their attitudes and accomplishments in academic areas. More-over, it will become clear that some of the attributes teachers find distasteful in children correspond to the characteristics they find trou-blesome in parents.

SCHOOLS, FAMILIES, AND DISTANCING

To extend the pupil–teacher relationship discussed earlier to the home–school relationship in regard to racial/ethnic attitudes, Lightfoot

(1981) argues that the development of boundaries and territoriality keeps parents and teachers (and other school officials) from meaningful relationships. She believes that territoriality exists because of racial attitudes and that schools organize public rituals such as PTA meetings, open houses, or newsletters that permit little true collaboration, negotiation, or criticism between parents and teachers. Interactions between these parties tend to be institutionalized ways for establishing boundaries under the pretense of polite cooperation. In working with minority families, territoriality must be lessened before true collaboration can occur.

In a related, large-scale study of 369 parents of children with mild disabilities, Arnold, Michael, Hosley, and Miller (in press) reported on parents who developed negative attitudes about communicating with the school in reaction to the school's attempt to provide special education information. In contrast, interactive activities between the school and family members led to positive attitudes relative to communicating with the schools.

Providing impersonal information (a distancing strategy) seemed to be a more comfortable way for the school to communicate than personal exchanges with family members. This reflects my opinion that at some level, school personnel believe that parents are a nuisance and that if allowed too close, they can be troublesome. In an effort to avoid interacting with parents, schools chose various distancing strategies. In turn, those forms of impersonal communication alienated parents from school staff, so that parents felt unwelcome, leading to negative views of schools and the professionals that populate them.

TEACHERS' ATTITUDES TOWARD PARENTS

I agree with Kaplan (1992), who wrote, "Parents are not the enemy. They care; they are concerned. It is the responsibility of the school to aggressively seek their cooperation, support and commitment" (p. 304).

Teachers' attitudes toward parents vary but tend to lean heavily toward the negative. Likewise, the attitudes of some parents toward teachers appear to be negative. In fact, dealing with parents has been cited as a stress-producing factor for educators and as a deterrent to job satisfaction (Pagel & Price, 1980; Smith & Cline, 1980). The first step in rectifying these attitudes is to be well informed about the underlying reasons for them and to consider whether they are rational or irrational.

As far as teachers are concerned, I suspect that a relationship exists between negative attitudes toward students and similar attitudes toward parents of children with disabilities. However, rather than finding these parents, per se, difficult to tolerate, teachers may harbor negative attitudes toward parents who manifest *attributes* similar to those of children they dislike. For different reasons, teachers may have negative attitudes toward aggressive children *and* parents, where the common denominator is aggressiveness and not the fact that they belong to the group "children" or "parents." Other factors that cut across group identities include speech, gender, socioeconomic status, perceived laziness (noncooperation), and cultural, national, or ethnic affiliation. Additionally, teachers' attitudes may be influenced by other characteristics regarded as deviations from the norm, for example, emotionally disturbed or mentally retarded parents, or parents who are public figures and/or professionals in the community.

In an excellent analysis of the teacher in society, Lortie (1975) uncovers the vulnerable position in which the teacher is often found. Teachers, Lortie asserts, have discernible reasons to distrust and even fear parents. In America, parents enjoy considerable rights in tending to the educational affairs of their children. Parents may and sometimes do complain to teachers or to administrative personnel about the teacher's performance. Repeated or serious complaints can have a deleterious effect on the teacher's standing within the school system. Lortie points out that teachers have the license to discipline children, but with conditions. Teachers who give vent to anger may fear parental sanctions, not the least of which is a lawsuit. Because of real or perceived threats, teachers do experience a sense of vulnerability that has its roots in reality.

Teachers are required to maintain a social order of democracy and fairness, as well as a viable instructional group, often under difficult circumstances. Lortie points out that parents who ask for special treatment for their child place the teacher in conflict, which is compounded when several parents make contradictory requests. The teacher is forced to choose between a philosophically democratic and fair social order and parental wishes for special attention. A barrage of parental requests makes teachers fear that their social order is beginning to unravel. To make matters worse, teachers are trying to sustain a social order with pupils over whom they have only limited authority.

Teachers are also dependent on parents in that they must rely on them to influence their children in ways that teachers value, namely to infuse a positive attitude toward schoolwork (Rutherford & Edgar,

1979; Lombana, 1983). Fears are generated by teachers' awareness that parental influence can range from sentiments of strong help and support to indifference or open hostility (Lortie, 1975). How parents choose to influence their children can have an important effect on the students' behavior in the classroom (Luszki & Schmuck, 1965), and studies have shown that when the values of the family and the school are contradictory, the students' schoolwork suffers (Shea & Bauer, 1991; Fox, Luszki, & Schmuck, 1966).

In one study, Lortie (1975) asked teachers about what they see as ideal parent–teacher relationships. In the study, teachers often depicted parent–teacher conferences as "a waste of time" or interpersonally awkward. Respondents wanted more contact with parents, but only when their children were having trouble in school. Eighty-eight percent of the teachers in the lower-status elementary schools wanted more contacts with parents, compared with 23% of teachers employed in higher-status schools. Parents in lower-status schools often failed to respond to teacher requests for a conference, whereas parents in the higher-status schools often showed up without invitation, a situation not to the liking of teachers.

Lortie's analysis suggests that the desired relationship places the teacher in the superordinate role, where the teacher defines occasions that justify parental involvement. Chronic, spontaneous visitors were characterized by teachers as "academic hypochondriacs worrying and fussing without cause." In other words, teacher-initiated conferences were looked upon favorably, but other parent visits were considered "interruptions."

Teachers' dependence on parents to motivate their child properly clashes with their wish to control the parent–teacher relationship. Even though teachers want to control the relationship, they do not have the status to make parents comply, making their vulnerability genuine. "The wish to control the workplace is combined with the wish for support from influential others—independence and dependence are contained in a formula based on boundedness and teacher initiation. The teacher's concerns are placed at the center of the ideal relationship; parents should comply with arrangements which meet teacher needs" (Lortie, 1975, p. 191).

From Lortie's research and analysis, we begin to gain some insight into the underlying causes of tension between parent and teacher. An added confounding influence is the principal. Teachers want to achieve autonomy from their superior yet require the principal's protection from overly intrusive parents. This situation throws the parent–

teacher–principal triad into a remarkably interlocking and potentially difficult system, with the teacher assuming the pivotal role—a role infused with contradictory needs and desires that require the teacher to choose between alternative resolutions of what must be a perplexing and tension-producing enigma. In this regard, Turnbull (1983) encourages parents to recognize the difficult position of some professionals. Although a strong advocate for parent rights, Turnbull believes that sometimes parents are unforgiving. Gargiulo (1985) appears to agree, asserting that family members sometimes condemn professionals for not recognizing the disability sooner and occasionally accuse the professional of causing the disability. Indeed, some parents inhibit the growth of their relationship with professionals by withdrawing or misjudging them to be insensitive, offensive, and incapable of understanding their situation (Seligman & Darling, 1997).

In asking teachers to describe the "good parent," Lortie reported that two central themes were reflected in the responses, namely, that parents should not intervene, and parents should support teachers' efforts. "Good parents" were characterized as "distant assistants" by imbuing the child with a positive attitude toward school, cooperating with the teacher yet not interfering, and taking the lead (direction) from the teacher.

Barsch (1969) observed that parents of children with disabilities accord the teacher a significantly more positive status than teachers accord parents: "Clinical experience with over 12,000 sets of parents and wide professional experience with many teachers confirm a belief that the parent is more favorable to the teacher than the teacher is to the parent" (p. 8). Bailard and Strang (1964) add that parents are appreciative of the genuine concern teachers show for their children, and Shapiro (1975) reports that good teachers are mentioned more often than any other factor when parents explain why their schools are good. He drew the following conclusions from his national survey examining parents' attitudes toward teachers:

> The lesson to be learned from the national survey data is that when people scan the universe to identify what is helping children's chances for a good life, they are more likely to identify schools than any other agent. Further, when asked to scan the universe to identify what might be hurting their children's chances for a good life, they are quite unlikely to identify schools. . . . (p. 270)

> If we can transmit [the public's] faith to beginning teachers, I believe they will feel free to function happily in their professional role, secure in their knowledge of the unique value that society accords them. (p. 273)

This paradox—where the teacher is negatively predisposed toward the parent and the parent is positively predisposed toward the teacher—is, according to Barsch (1969), at the root of many of the problems reflected in negative school–parent encounters.

Moreover, parents and teachers differ in their perception of the child. To the teacher, he is one member of the category "student," and to the parent he is a special, prized person. Special considerations for a child, which are sometimes asked of the teacher and emerge from the parents' vantage point that their child is unique and deserving of special attention, run counter to the teacher's perception that the child is just another pupil.

Adding to the growth of unfortunate stereotypes is the belief that parents fall into the same general categories as their children; that is, parents of children with physical disabilities are somehow different than parents of children who are mentally retarded, and so on. Barsch's (1968) study of child-rearing practices among parents of five different disability populations failed to substantiate the belief that there are significant differences among parents that can be attributed simply to the exceptionality of their children.

Along the same line, Bissell (1976) argues that parents are dehumanized by categorical references and generalizations. Parents tend to be cast into two discrete groups: those with normal children, and those with children who have disabilities. These stereotypes of parents tend to be quite prevalent and surprising at a time when educators are endorsing prescriptive, individualized, noncategorical approaches to education, especially in the education of exceptional children. In referring to his own experiences, Bissell comments:

> [My] initial high levels of anxiety related to a perception of these parents as pathological [which] did not enhance the probability of establishing a climate of positive mutual regard and effective communication. Only through experience was [I] able to learn that each parent is a unique developing individual, and [my] helping efforts were maximized as [I] became able to discard negative perceptions. The cliches and myths about exceptional parents and techniques for *handling* them were minimized by real experiences with parents as persons. (p. 219)

Teachers may generally feel threatened by professionals, who are perceived as better educated, more intelligent, or pillars of the community. Being in awe of well-known or highly educated parents of children with exceptionality is not uncommon, but the teacher should keep in mind that these people have the same strengths, repertoire of coping mechanisms, and similar vulnerabilities as other parents, and at times require a teacher's expert counsel about schooling and parenting issues.

Parents are frequently viewed by teachers from a pathological perspective (i.e., in terms of making maladaptive adjustments to their children), a reality that can be attributed in part to the sometimes pathological way parents are characterized in the professional literature (Seligman & Seligman, 1980; Simpson, 1996). In some cases, parents are not viewed as desirable or competent full-fledged members of the interdisciplinary team because their perceptions of their own child are regarded as negligible or, even more negative, as a distortion of reality. Parents are often considered a nuisance rather than a resource and are frequently criticized, analyzed, or made to feel responsible for their child's problems. It is not unusual to hear teachers call parents lazy and stupid, demanding, greedy, conniving, or angry and defensive (Rubin & Quinn-Curran, 1983). Furthermore, research has shown that professionals (not just education professionals) increase feelings of guilt, confusion, and frustration in family members (Bernheim & Lehman, 1985). On the other hand, teachers tend to view parents as more capable when they have more frequent interactions (Michael, Arnold, Magliocca, & Miller, 1992, cited in Turnbull, 1983). This finding suggests that face-to-face meetings between parents and teachers can contribute to positive collaborative relationships.

The emergence of parent organizations can be viewed as a threat to the teacher; they are seen as enemies having tremendous resources and presenting realistic dangers. For some professionals, parents have traditionally been viewed as adversaries rather than allies (Carberry, 1975; Losen & Diament, 1978).

Parent organizations have grown in popularity, and it is a fact that some of these groups have acted assertively in contributing to positive changes in school programs and, hence, opportunities for children with disabilities. Parent groups have been a major force in influencing legislative efforts in the interest of their children (Simpson, 1996). Most groups have been formed for mutual self-help and are not designed to threaten or cajole anyone, much less the teachers whom parents admire and on whom they rely (Seligman, 1991).

There are teachers who, not threatened by such groups, show a sincere desire to work cooperatively with parents and voluntarily attend parent meetings. The interchange that takes place allows the parent to ask educationally relevant questions of the teacher and enables the teacher to learn about the mechanisms of peer self-help groups and gain a more intimate understanding of the problems parents experience. Perhaps the most important gain is the parents' perception that teachers care and know that parents can be their allies.

A publication by the Council for Exceptional Children (undated) notes that it is little wonder why some teachers are afraid to talk to parents. A child's parents tend to be thought of as "problems" with which the teacher must contend. Some teachers believe that others who have worked with the child and/or the parents contribute to their current problems. Unconsciously, or consciously, teachers may blame parents for causing a child's problems or, at least, for not having prevented them.

Just like counselors who on occasion are assigned clients they have difficulty accepting, teachers may find themselves in a similar position with parents. Unlike social service agencies, where a transfer of a client can be made to another counselor or social worker, the teacher finds herself in a less flexible position. In such instances, the teacher might try to examine what she and the parents each contribute to their problematic relationship. She can be introspective about the relationship or discuss it with a supervisor or colleague. It is important to keep in mind, however, that the teacher has the most control over her own emotions and behavior, not those of the parents.

While recognizing that some parental attributes are difficult to accept, a teacher may wish to consider some of the positive characteristics of parents and try to respond to and reinforce these in parent–teacher conferences, while ignoring their negative characteristics to whatever extent possible. Teachers faced with a difficult parent situation should always have the opportunity to confer with a colleague or supervisor. In some cases, third-party objectivity can help.

Teachers are often asked to assume several different roles in relation to parents (Simpson, 1996; Reynolds & Birch, 1977; Schulz, 1987). These additional roles augment the pedagogical role they have traditionally held and include supervising parent aides, evaluating student progress and conveying the information to parents, working with parents on school policy and in developing community activities, and acting as the child's "parent" during the school day. To these roles one might add that teachers should assume responsibility for making appropriate referrals and facilitating good student–student relationships, dealing with parents and siblings of children with disabilities, and being proficient in class management, among other skills (Reynolds, Birch, Grohs, Howsam, & Morsink, 1980). Ayers (1986) believes that teachers should also help to empower parents and families, help them take control of their circumstances, and support them in making decisions with regard to their children. Citing the work of Dunst and Trivette, Shea and Bauer (1991) observed that "in the most effective interactions, the helping teacher assumes a positive stance toward the parents and families; emphasizes the role and responsibilities of the family for solving their problems and meeting their needs; assumes that the families with whom they are working have the capacity to understand, learn and manage events in their lives; and builds on strengths rather than attempting to remediate problems" (pp. 49–50).

In summary, Ayers (1986) feels that effective teachers need to interact conscientiously with parents and make themselves available to them. Whether teachers assume all these roles, some of them, or take on other responsibilities, it is obvious that additional tasks and pressures have been placed on them in recent years. In authoritarian, nonsupportive climates, teachers may react strongly against assuming added responsibility—an attitude that ultimately affects their relationships with students and parents. In supportive settings, people tend to work cooperatively toward productive ends. As mentioned earlier, administrative support is essential (Lambie & Daniels-Mohring, 1993; Meyan et al., 1996). In any case, overwhelming burdens and pressures, and a poor school climate may contribute to teachers' negative reactions to parents. In such instances, parents may be seen as an added pressure, consuming inordinate amounts of time and energy—resources that teachers feel they can ill afford.

> Educators find themselves in a psychological squeeze. They are required to be more "accountable" for the effectiveness of programs; they are subject to pressures by local communities and by state and federal attempts to establish standards of quality and equality. At the same time, they find themselves increasingly burdened with responsibility for basic socialization for children, and experience frustration, discouragement, and anger over what they view as an abdication of responsibility by parents. (Hetznecker, 1978, p. 364)

To this Corrigan and Howey (1980) add:

> Society now demands a new breed of teacher for a new breed of school—a well prepared, highly motivated professional, capable of understanding a broad range of learning problems and of designing and implementing curricular and instructional strategies to solve them. If the school of the future is to become a vehicle for social prog-

ress then a sense of social purpose must pervade every level of the educational system and the teaching profession. (p. 211)

Parents have a mix of positive and negative emotions toward their
child with a disability and the teacher should be accepting of these
contradictory, yet normal, human feelings. Although teachers may
find burdensome a parent's gloomy outlook, ambivalent feelings, or
occasional acute bouts of depression over their circumstances, it is important for them to recognize and allow for contradictory feelings and
actions, and not regard them as "bad" or abnormal. Our culture
guards well the reality that *all* parents harbor mixed feelings about
their children, fostering the myth that feelings should be positive at all
times.

Teachers' attitudes toward parents are not as healthy as they
should be. The combined factors of working with challenging children
and parents; added roles, pressures, and responsibilities that teachers
have been asked to assume; unsupportive work environments; and
negative cognitions about parents that have developed over the years
result in attitudes and behaviors that impede rather than facilitate rapport between parents and teachers. Concerted efforts must be made by
school personnel to recognize this situation, and supervisors and educators must develop (in college and university teacher-training programs and in-service meetings) strategies that will change it.

The threat that parents represent to teachers is reflected in a study
showing that elementary teachers found parents to be particularly
challenging and frustrating to beginning teachers (Houston & Wil-
liamson, 1990, cited in Kaplan, 1992, p. 257). Virtually all of the 42 que-
ried teachers mentioned such concerns as uncooperative parents, uninvolved parents, noncompliant parents, and the like. These teachers
said that preservice content relating to relationships with parents and
conferencing with them were covered poorly, if at all, in their university and college programs. Houston and Houston (1992) add:

> Preparing prospective teachers to be knowledgeable about parent-
> conferences is too low an expectation for effective teacher preparation
> programs. The influence of the family on the child is too great to ig-
> nore. Simply having the skills to conduct parent conferences does not
> go beyond technical competence to tap the essence of professional
> preparation. The psycho/sociological influence of the family is com-
> manding and powerful. It deserves to be placed in its proper perspec-
> tive in the study of culture and society in education as well as the tech-
> niques of parent-conferences. (p. 257)

The first step, then, is accepting the existence of untoward attitudes. Recognition of a problem generally provides the insight and impetus or motivation for subsequent change. The second step is the implementation of strategies designed to modify attitudes—admittedly not an easy task, but one that must be undertaken. The exercises included in this volume should prove helpful toward this end.

TEACHERS' ATTITUDES TOWARD CHANGE

The field of education has embarked on a challenging venture, namely, the appropriate education of children with disabilities in regular public school classrooms (Simpson, 1996; Turnbull & Turnbull, 1986; Turnbull, Turnbull, Shank, & Leal, 1995). This trend has implications for special as well as regular education schoolteachers and is being met with a mixed response. As with other innovations in education, the teacher is rarely consulted or considered but is merely informed of anticipated changes and required to attend workshops in which the new ideology or methodology is expounded. The general disregard for the sentiment or opinion of the teacher, combined with a tendency for people in general to resist major changes in their personal or professional lives, has major implications for how current mandated changes will be carried out.

The resistance and challenge connected with the inclusion of children with exceptionalities in public schools require immediate and intensive study. This problem has become particularly acute since the passage of Public Law 94-142 (the Education for All Handicapped Children Act), which reinforces our national commitment to a free and appropriate education for every child with a disability. Attitudes toward new ideologies and programs have a direct bearing on their effectiveness when they are implemented. Thus, how regular schoolteachers feel about having children with disabilities in their classrooms, and how special education teachers view their changing roles, are areas that should be subject to investigation now and in the coming years. They certainly should be topics for discussion in classrooms in colleges and universities.

In realizing constructive attitudinal change toward new programs, it is imperative that we do not follow the same unproductive practices used in attempts to change teachers' attitudes toward student characteristics. The brief workshop model falls far short of achieving fundamental changes in ideology and behavior. Successful implementation of organizational changes is a gradual, long-term process in which the new ideology and its accompanying strategies are the subject of ongoing interaction, not administrative edict. Important in this process of accommodation to new programs is the opportunity for teachers to communicate their opinions and express their views without threat and be given the chance to provide input into new and developing programs. The likelihood of success of new programs and positive teacher attitudes are immeasurably greater if the school administration is supportive and provides a positive model for staff and faculty (Stern & Keislar, 1977; Schulz, 1987; Meyan et al., 1996). Administrative support of parent involvement in the schools is so important that it bears repeating. Some time ago, Glass (1969) advised that "one of the important factors of getting parents into the school is to develop a climate within the school—that is, within the faculty—that will be favorable towards the parents, an atmosphere that will encourage parents to participate. The development of this climate is the responsibility of the administrator and his representatives" (p. 167).

It is essential to recognize that beliefs, attitudes, and behavior developed over many years do not dissipate by mandate but may be altered over time and under conducive circumstances. Actually, attitudinal changes toward alterations in organizations or programs appear more likely and easier to accomplish than firmly held attitudes toward other people.

> With reference to the general issue of effecting teacher attitude change, it should be pointed out that even in the most strongly held beliefs about organization, methods, and content of instruction, there is far less resistance to modification than when deep-seated emotional feelings are tapped. Attitudes toward children from different religious and racial groups, from different cultures and environments, are based on the teachers' own life-time history of conditioning and are far more impervious to short-term, superficial training modes. (Stern & Keislar, 1977, p. 73)

PARENTS' ATTITUDES TOWARD TEACHERS

We recall Barsch's (1969) observation that teachers view parents more negatively than parents view teachers. Although parents have made complaints about and hold negative attitudes toward professionals in general, teachers tend to be spared such negative evaluations from parents. This is not to say that parents' attitudes toward teachers are uniformly positive, as the following discussion reveals.

Rowe (1978) hypothesizes that unconscious transference occurs in the parents' relationships to the professional. For example, parents may transfer feelings they still have for important (especially authority) figures in their childhood. Some parents, seeing the teacher as a parent, may try to take the role of the dependent child by trying to please or placate her. Conversely, parents may present themselves to teachers with an unconsciously rebellious or hostile attitude that is really an expression of unresolved feelings for their own parents or their schooling experience. Orlosky (1992, cited in Kaplan, 1992, p. 141) reminds us that conferences take place on the teachers turf. Although now the turf of their children, a parent's presence in a school environment is a reminder of earlier experiences with teachers and other school personnel.

> Underneath most parents is a student—someone who went to school, sometimes happily, sometimes unhappily. What often happens when the parent-as-adult returns to school, or has dealings with teachers, is that the parent as child/student returns. Many parents still enter school buildings flooded with old memories, angers, and disappointments. Their stomachs churn and flutter with butterflies, not because of what is happening today with their own children, but because of outdated memories and past behaviors. (Rich, 1987, cited in Kaplan, 1992, p. 155)

Also, parents may view teachers solely as imparters of information to children and may, therefore, balk at scheduled parent–teacher conferences. If teachers are seen only in this role, parents could well be puzzled by comments they make about the child's emotional responses and classroom behavior. Such narrow perceptions of a teacher's role generally diminishes as the parent gains a clearer perception of a teacher's multifaceted responsibilities; most parents probably would find considerable comfort in knowing that the teacher is keenly aware of their child's development from more than just an academic point of view.

Some parents' perceptions are colored by unfortunate professional encounters in the past. These parents will approach the teacher with caution to see if prior experiences will be repeated. Such parents will be relieved and able to change their preconceived attitudes in the company of a facilitative ally. In regard to parental expectations, mothers of children with severe disabilities were asked to share their expectations of professionals (Schulz, 1987). The most frequently expressed expectations were honesty, respect, and empathy. Several mothers had expectations that professionals should make an effort to see the child from their perspective and to have genuine affection for the child.

Teachers may be seen by parents as competitors if the values they emphasize do not coincide with the parents' own (Lortie, 1975). In such an instance, parents may feel undercut in their efforts to raise their child, and they envy the teacher who excites the child's affection and respect. This reaction may be particularly true of parents whose sole source of emotional gratification is their child. If the teacher senses competition for the child's attention from the parents, the issue should be addressed as soon as possible. During conferences, a teacher might mention the child's comments about his parents or objects he made for them (birthday or holiday gifts) to reinforce the critical role they play in his life. It might be well to point out that children tend to talk about their teachers in their parents' presence, and that it is not uncommon for the child to speak proudly of his parents to his teacher. Another possibility is to encourage involvement of the parents in the child's education, thereby decreasing their feelings of competition.

As mentioned earlier, the parent–teacher relationship as well as student learning are greatly enhanced when parents convey to their children positive attitudes toward school (Shea & Bauer, 1991). Conversely, parents who have bitter memories of school and communicate their unsympathetic attitudes to their children can have an adverse effect: "Memories of authoritarian teachers, strict administrators, and drab surroundings influence their attitudes toward the school" (Schulz, 1987, p. 148).

Unrealistic views of the teacher's ability could result in parental demands and expectations the teacher is unprepared and unable to fulfill. Teachers may be perceived as counselors and psychotherapists, capable of dispensing advice about significant psychological problems, or as clergymen or attorneys of sorts, qualified to advise about religious or legal matters. There will be times when teachers are in a position to provide support and comfort, and occasions will arise when direct advice is appropriate, but teachers should be careful to stay within the boundaries of their competency.

Age-old concerns about proper child-rearing practices may emerge as parents come to know the teacher's style of interaction with children. Methods of discipline that the parent practices at home will probably be the ones the parent wishes to see the teacher use in school. Permissive parents may be appalled by the teacher's use of what they consider to be harsh disciplinary methods, whereas strict parents will be puzzled by the permissiveness with which their child is treated at school. In either case, the teacher should be prepared to explain to the parent the potential benefit of his approach. This effort should lessen the parents' concern, as they will then view the teacher as one who has a well-thought-out strategy and is willing to share it, thereby opening the channels of communication and forming the basis for dialogue and mutual respect. Teachers should be careful of believing that withholding information from parents is a sign of professionalism.

In their sincere desire to motivate parents to help their child, teachers may make impossible demands that can cause discouragement and despair. Insensitivity to the resources of the parents and family is counterproductive. The overburdening of parents is generally done inadvertently but the effects of conscientious working parents attempting to respond to the demands of several professionals can lead to excessive stress and create family problems (Seligman & Darling, 1997). Especially in instances of severe childhood disability where a number of professionals are involved, the teacher may wish to inquire about what tasks have been assigned by others working with the child/family. Ideally, some families could benefit from a person who serves as "coordinator of services" to help monitor the multifaceted demands sometimes made on parents (Laborde & Seligman, 1991).

Teachers should maintain an awareness of how they may be perceived by the parents. Parents may, for example, react with anxiety and begin to develop negative attitudes toward the teacher as a result of a previous meeting. It is difficult for a teacher to know how a particular comment will be received, although sensitive teachers with good interpersonal skills rarely make potentially destructive comments. Nevertheless, a teacher may have inadvertently and without malice touched upon a particularly sensitive area or made a comment that was misconstrued. In either event, a change in the parents' typical way of interacting may signal that something has gone amiss. The teacher should make an inquiry at this point instead of waiting until negative attitudes or feelings become more intransigent and it becomes increasingly difficult for either the teacher or the parents to broach the issue.

It is important to make the distinction between parents who knew early of the child's exceptionality and have become accommodated to the situation and parents who are just beginning to realize their child's limitations. Such dawning awareness is not necessarily a reflection of denial now giving way to reality but of the emergence of more obvious manifestations of impaired development not apparent during earlier years.

Although professionals must allow for individualized expressions of anxiety and stress, the teacher might expect the "accommodated" parents to be less questioning, less fearful, less confused, and probably more confident than the parents still adjusting to the child's disability. The latter may require more support from the teacher as well as honest and understanding responses to their questions.

Being aware of the parents' position in the denial–acceptance continuum should help professionals anticipate feelings and behaviors that correspond to a particular stage and respond to them accordingly. This behavior should predispose parents to view teachers in a more positive fashion. By the same token, teachers must be aware that their best predictions may turn out to be wrong and that they must remain open to unanticipated experiences.

Negative parental attitudes may not be directed toward the teacher but reflect what the *conference* may mean to the parent. As mentioned previously, negative meetings with other professionals predispose parents to anticipate that subsequent conferences will deal only with the child's weaknesses—deficiencies that are painfully apparent and that the parent does not wish to have validated by still another professional. There will probably be more cooperation from parents and better attendance at conferences if they are balanced to reflect both their child's strengths and deficiencies. The teacher should try not to barrage parents of significantly impaired children with a laundry list of problems. Such conferences can have a devastating effect on the parent psychologically and destroy whatever rapport the parents and teacher may have developed. One parent describes her experience at a team meeting thusly:

> My confidence ebbs away as I sit, outnumbered ten to one, at a conference table full of "professionals." These people speak in low, assured tones, one after another, and I listen, bewildered, to: Woodcock, WISC, Matrix Analogies, scores, indicated strengths and needs, projected start dates, short-term instructional objectives. Everyone nods and smiles. I sign here, initial there, and am ushered out. I cry in the car before I start the engine. Where is my child in all this data?
>
> I wish for one person, who knows my child, who cares deeply about his daily experiences as well as his future, someone who understands the terminology and the options and could be useful in such a meeting. These professionals wanted what was correct, cer-

tainly, but they also wanted expediency. Who would protect my child in all of this; who would help him achieve the vision that we have for him? (in Bradley et al., 1997, pp. 168–169)

In team meetings where other professionals may be present (e.g., school psychologist, social worker, occupational therapist, speech therapist), special efforts must be made to keep the conference in perspective. Because hearing about the child's limitations from each of the professionals represented at the meeting may be more than some parents can endure, the meetings must be conducted with sensitivity and good judgment. The communication of negative or delicate material should be done on a one-to-one basis, allowing parents to meet with someone with whom rapport has been established. During meetings, it is important to allow parents time to ask questions and to offer their perceptions.

Parents who have had lifelong problems with authority figures may have negative attitudes toward the teacher before they ever meet. The anxiety generated by conferring with yet another authority (in this case, the teacher) could result in one of two possible reactions: taking the offensive (e.g., directing angry remarks to the teacher) or withdrawing (e.g., not attending scheduled parent–teacher conferences). In the first instance, the parents' anxiety and anger should diminish in the presence of a professional who does not reciprocate in kind. In the second, the parents' courage may be summoned by a teacher who, perhaps more than once, warmly invites them to meet with her.

The parent–teacher relationship is greatly improved when both parents are present at the conference. In this way, both mother and father are involved, and the chances for distortion of what occurred during the conference are minimized. Granted, gender roles are less rigid now than in the past; however, in many families, the mother is still considered the one who is responsible for the basic needs of the children. Therefore, the teacher should not be surprised if only the mother attends the conference. Every effort should be made, however, to encourage fathers to attend conferences.

It should be noted that a father's reluctance to attend a conference may be more related to anxieties about the child than a reflection of male behavior. In fact, some fathers use the coping strategy of distancing when they have anxieties about their child with a disability (Houser & Seligman, 1991; Meyer, 1995). Even so, the teacher should make an effort to involve fathers. For some fathers, all that is needed is to schedule a conference time after working hours.

Gently urging the parent to bring her spouse to a conference where their child is discussed is to be encouraged. But if the teacher senses that there is considerable resistance, the matter should be dropped, at least temporarily. Although some teachers may rail at the rather stereotypical and rigid role behavior manifested in some families, it is essential that the parents' lifestyle and role structure, as well as their culture, be respected.

Special consideration should be given to the single-parent exceptional family (Seligman & Darling, 1997). Reliance on the teacher for support and help may be heavy because, of necessity, single parents must assume greater responsibility for themselves and their offspring. Also, the single-parent structure is growing, yet is still a minority one with which our society is ill equipped to deal effectively. The minority status of being a single parent is compounded by that of being a parent of a child with a disability—a dual burden that can be overwhelming psychologically.

Foster parents and adoptive parents might hold attitudes toward the teacher similar to those discussed in this chapter, but their special relationship to their children may generate challenges of a slightly different nature. For example, foster parents generally keep the child for a circumscribed period of time; thus, the parents' involvement may be more marginal. On the whole, foster parents genuinely care for the children they accept into their family. However, the teacher should be watchful of neglectful foster parents whose motive to provide a home for the child is more closely related to monetary gain than genuine affection.

Although it is not always the case, usually, parents who voluntarily accept a child with a disability into the family do so with considerable knowledge of the problems that lie ahead. Such parents should prove to be cooperative and helpful. In terms of the self-reported needs of foster parents, Noble and Euster (1981) found that over half of the surveyed parents wanted to know more about child management and communication with their foster children. Another study of foster parents of children with disabilities reported that they spent twice as much money as other foster parents, especially for equipment (Arkava & Mueller, 1976).

Some negative attitudes seemingly directed toward teachers have little to do with either the teacher, the school, or the conference per se. Parents may feel intimidated by the educational discrepancy between themselves and the teacher; as a result, they may approach the conference with a feeling of inferiority. This may cause parents to be less open during conferences. However, as the parent–teacher relationship evolves, parents tend to feel more comfortable in the teacher's presence as they sense his nonjudgmental attitude. Skillful teachers who can communicate a feeling of positive regard irrespective of the parents' personal qualities eventually gain the trust of the people with whom they work. It should be noted that positive regard that is expressed unconditionally (that is, no matter what the person's attributes) is an important characteristic for helping professionals to acquire. It may be learned over time, but it is easier to have positive, accepting feelings toward others if one has internalized early the philosophy that people who are different in certain ways have worth. In this sense, unconditional positive regard is more a component of one's personality than an easily acquired skill.

Age differences initially may be viewed by parents in a negative manner. A recently graduated young teacher conferring with older parents may cause both parties some consternation during the first few conferences. However, the teacher's rapport with the parents, as well as the demonstration of her expertise, will reduce any concerns about age differences. In rare instances, parents may continue to regard a young or young-appearing teacher as a "learned daughter." Actually, this perception is not at all negative, as long as the parent remains cooperative and the primary focus is on the child's development.

Interestingly, age differences can constitute more of a problem for the teacher than the parents. Perceiving the parent as older and more knowledgeable can be a source of difficulty for the teacher. In countertransference* terms, some teachers may view and react to the parent as they responded to their harsh and demanding mothers or fathers, especially if the parent possesses similar characteristics and mannerisms. A helpful strategy for teachers is to continually separate, at a cognitive level, the child's parents from their own parents. The teacher might say (to himself) something like, "Although they

---

*Not only can a parent transfer conflicts with past figures onto the relationships with the teacher, but the teacher does likewise with the parent. These feelings are called countertransference. Ideally, the teacher should be totally aware of them, so that they do not interfere with the relationship. The negative aspect of countertransference occurs when the teacher is not able to understand the parent objectively because of his own conflicts and needs. But by monitoring the feelings the parent elicits in him, the teacher can often gain an understanding of the conflicts facing the parent and thus can better appreciate how the parent affects other people.

are older and have some similar characteristics [to my father/ mother], they are, after all, *not* my parents but people who have come to me, a professional." Because such countertransference is sometimes resistant to change, professional psychotherapists are required during their training to engage in personal therapy, so that previous reactions to significant others do not interfere with their efforts to help their clients.

In regard to discipline, not only can parents and teachers differ in their perceptions of proper disciplinary strategies, but also each party may experience different "truths" about a particular child (Hetznecker, Arnold, & Phillips, 1978). Chances are, parents and teacher are both right and wrong. However, ritualized, time-limited conferences do not allow for a productive exchange leading to perceptual modifications, compromise, and a more accurate and comprehensive picture of the child. A richer perspective can be obtained if the teacher learns more about the child at home and the parents learn more about the child in the classroom. Different perceptions of the child need not end in controversy but should culminate in a fuller and richer understanding of the child's world, which encompasses more than just school or home.

In their efforts to get parents more interested and involved, teachers and principals may launch an aggressive program to achieve better home–school relationships. Such attitudes and enthusiasm can hardly be criticized, yet a few precautions are necessary. Overeager teachers may actually generate negative attitudes if parents feel pressured into greater school involvement or more frequent parent–teacher conferences. However, negative feelings generally stem from the way in which parents are approached. Frequent notices brought home by the child, "reminder" phone calls, or letters mailed to the parents should be avoided. Notes or letters should only be sent occasionally and written in a way that would allow parents to feel invited but not coerced or made to feel guilty. The same is true of phone calls. Any invitations should have a purpose and must be communicated to parents before the conference.

Conversely, school personnel may become disheartened if they perceive that their enthusiastic effort born of genuine concern has seemingly reaped few benefits. Too often, excessive enthusiasm leads to rather grandiose expectations and then discouragement. Too much is anticipated too soon. School personnel should savor the gains they have made, whether large or small, and build on what has been accomplished. Poorly learned by many professionals is the lesson that

change in the attitudes and behaviors of human beings is often painfully slow.

Parents' perception of teachers, the school, or schooling constitute
a varied tapestry of attitudes and expectations. On the whole, parents
tend to value their child's teacher as one who is generally knowledgeable, a specialist in educating children, and a source of encouragement
and support. With the exception of a minority of parents with whom it
is difficult to work, they constitute a formidable ally for the teacher in
the teaching–learning enterprise.

3

Family Dynamics:
An Overview

$\mathbf{B}$y understanding family dynamics, teachers and other school personnel can make realistic appraisals of the child with a disability and his family, the family's burdens, their coping mechanisms, and the strengths that sustain them. Also, such knowledge helps the teacher understand parental reactions that might otherwise appear to be strange, unreasonable, and at times, incomprehensible. Families come in numerous forms, from the conventional married couple with children to divorced parents, single parents, and gay parents.

Ethnicity and Family Therapy, edited by McGoldrick, Giordano, and Pearce (1996), now in its second edition, is considered a classic in the field of multiculturalism and the family, and covers the unique attributes of persons from numerous cultural, racial, and ethnic origins. For McGoldrick and Giordano (1996), in an overview chapter of this book, the definition of what constitutes a family goes beyond married, divorced, single, or gay parents. It incorporates how cultural affiliations alter the meaning of "family":

> The dominant American (Anglo) definition focuses on the intact nuclear family, whereas African-American families focus on a much wider network of kin and community. For Italians, there is no such

thing as the "nuclear" family. To them, family means a strong, tightly knit third- or fourth-generational network, which also includes godparents and old friends. The Chinese include in " family" all their ancestors and all their descendants, which also reflects a different sense of time than is held in the West. (p. 10)

McGoldrick and Giordano (1996) also discuss in some detail family attributes that reflect individuals' cultural heritage. They believe that professionals need to understand unique family characteristics to help them appreciate the richness of family life. This knowledge should also help professionals consider their own biases that may interfere with constructive relationships. As McGoldrick and Giordano contend:

> Certain common ethnic traits have been described as typical for families of one or another group. For example, Jewish families are often seen as valuing education, success, family connections, encouragement of children, democratic principles, verbal expression, shared suffering, and having a propensity to guilt and a love for eating. Anglos has been characterized as generally emphasizing control, personal responsibility, independence, individuality, stoicism, keeping up appearances, and moderation in everything. By contrast, Italian American families are generally described as valuing the family more than the individual; considering food a major source of emotional as well as physical nourishment; and having strong traditional male–female roles, with loyalty flowing through personal relationships. African Americans are often described as favoring an informal kinship network and spiritual values. Their strength to survive is a powerful resource, and they tend to have more flexibility in family roles than many other groups. In Hispanic cultures, family togetherness and respect, especially for elders, are valued concepts. People are appreciated more for their character than for merely their vocational success. They may also hold on to traditional notions of a woman's role as the virgin and the sacrificial sainted mother, who tolerates her husband's adventures and absence with forebearance. Chinese families stress harmony and interdependence in relationships, respect for one's place in the line of generations, ancestor worship, saving face, and food as an emotional and spiritual expression. For Asian Indians, purity, sacrifice, passivity, and a spiritual orientation are core values and death is seen as just one more phase in the life cycle that includes many rebirths.
>
> It would require many volumes to consider any single ethnic group in depth. Indeed, most groups are themselves combinations of multiple cultural groups. (p. 10)

Families coping with a member who has a chronic illness or disability are receiving increased attention (Moos, 1984; Rolland, 1993; Seligman & Darling, 1997; Marshak & Seligman, 1993; Ramsey, 1989; McDaniel, Hepworth, & Doherty, 1992). This "difference in the family," a phrase from a book title by Helen Featherstone (1980), can affect the family in numerous ways. This chapter explores some key concepts in family systems theory to provide a foundation for the central focus in this book, namely, the understanding of childhood disability in the family.

Just as a physical insult to the body or a severe psychological shock or trauma, such as rape or incest, can impede an individual's development, an event of major proportions can have a similar effect on the family. Families, like individuals, progress through various developmental stages, and many interacting factors help fashion a family's response to events—a response that may interfere with normal family development (Walsh, 1993). Also, the family unit is not a singular entity reacting as one to external stimuli but an interacting, interdependent group of individuals. An event that affects one member also either directly or indirectly affects the others:

> One image of the family that conveys its interconnectedness is that of the mobile. Like a huge cast steel Calder mobil, or a small one hanging over a baby's crib, each piece in the structure is connected to every other. Movement in one part of the mobile necessarily sets off change in each other part until the entire structure inevitably reestablishes a balance, a homeostasis, and comes to rest. It may be useful to think of this family as structured like a mobile, set in motion by a shift from within or without, seeking a balance appropriate for its particular structure, while needing to be flexible and capable of movement. (Elman, 1991, p. 370)

Moreover, the family is not a closed group, existing in isolation, but an open system relating to other such systems in the environment (Imber-Black, 1988; Bronfenbrenner, 1979; Seligman & Darling, 1997).

Role changes may affect a family unit, and altered roles are brought about by certain events that impinge on family life. Consider how family roles may be altered as a consequence of the following events:

1. The first baby born to a couple
2. Father laid off from work and mother forced to secure a job for financial reasons

3. Coddled daughter greeted by demanding newborn sibling
4. Divorce—impact on both parents and children
5. Death of a father or mother
6. Grandparent joining (living with) the family

In addition to social roles, other important aspects of family dynamics include decision-making processes, dominance behavior, conflict resolution, social behavior, social status, and the need for upward mobility (Turner, 1970). In complex ways, these factors influence how a significant event will be perceived and dealt with in the family. It is predicted that an event of some magnitude (e.g., the birth of a newborn with a disability) will contribute to the modification of certain family roles and dynamics.

SOCIAL ROLES

An important aspect of family dynamics is the notion of social roles, defined as a goal-directed pattern or sequence of acts tailored by cultural processes for the transactions a person may carry out in his or her social group (in this case the family) (Spiegel, 1957). Each position involves roles relative to other positions in the network as determined by cultural expectations and values. For example, a mother enacts certain roles and is held to certain role expectations by her children and husband. A family's functions tend to become differentiated into several often complementary roles (Raven & Rubin, 1976). For example, one family member may assume the role of "social smoother" by attempting to settle arguments between family members, while another member may take the role of "decision maker." Such roles are not formally designated but are more subtly derived. When the need arises, the family may expect a member to assume the role that has become expected. The subtlety and rigidity of family roles has been described by Kundera (1980) thusly:

> Every love relationship is based on unwritten conventions rashly agreed upon by the lovers during the first weeks of their love. On the one hand, they're living a sort of dream. On the other, without realizing it, they are drawing up the fine print of their contracts like the most hardnosed of lawyers. Old lovers! Be wary during those perilous first days! If you serve the other party breakfast in bed, you will be obliged to continue the same in perpetuity or face charges of animosity and treason! (p. 36)

The fluidity of roles that increasingly characterizes society today makes role expectations more difficult to predict, yet role flexibility is an essential characteristic of families facing childhood disability (Rolland, 1993).

As noted, social roles do not exist in isolation but tend to complement the role of someone else or fit into the role structure of a group (or family).

> As long as the role each family member occupies is complementary with and conforms to the role expectations other members have for him, the family lives in dynamic equilibrium. As soon as a discrepancy occurs, however—that is, when two or more family members have conflicting or incompatible notions on how to play their reciprocal roles—complementarity fails and the role system moves toward disequilibrium. Such disequilibrium is experienced by the family members in the form of tension, anxiety, hostility, or self-consciousness and individuals will try to deal with these reactions in a variety of ways. (Ross, 1964, p. 7)

COPING MECHANISMS

An understanding of how human beings cope with stressful situations represents an important dimension for understanding families with a child who has a disability. Defense mechanisms or coping mechanisms are "the means by which the organism protects itself against impulses and threats" (Hensie & Campbell, 1970, p. 182). The *American Psychiatric Glossary* (1988) defines defense mechanisms as "unconscious intrapsychic processes serving to provide relief from emotional conflict and anxiety" (p. 45). To put it another way, defense mechanisms help one to cope with excessive anxiety. Anna Freud (1948) discussed in some detail the defense mechanisms in common use today. It is of some importance to note that these mechanisms sometimes serve in a positive way to lessen anxiety; at other times, they interfere with an objective appraisal of a situation or event and, therefore, hamper its resolution. The double-edged nature of defense (or coping) mechanisms against anxiety becomes clearer in the following discussion.

Situations that generate unacceptable impulses or anxiety are sometimes perceived as having their source outside the self. The coping mechanism that projects blame onto an external source is called *projection*, in which an action or behavior is attributed to another person, group, or institution. It also reflects the tendency to attribute to others those aspects of oneself that one personally denies having

(Seligman & Rosenhan, 1998). Ross (1964) explains that the use of projection by parents of children with disabilities, by thrusting blame for the child's condition onto external sources, is a defense against unconscious guilt. The unconscious guilt may be related to realistic or unrealistic factors that the parents believe are related to the child's disability. The physician may be the object of the projection, or the source of blame may be something less tangible, such as heredity or a certain belief system. The frustration of not being able to pin a child's exceptionality on a particular cause allows it to be ascribed to a host of causes and results in fantasies about the probable cause or whether it could have been prevented (Hollingsworth & Pasnaw, 1977).

In looking for someone to blame, parents may blame each other, a grandparent, the school, or the teacher, although doctors make convenient scapegoats, especially during the infant and early childhood years. Teachers, the educational system, or other institutions may be more common projections as the child grows older. Unconscious guilt on the parents' part, for example, over not spending more time with a child or not finding time to help with academic subjects, may be converted into blaming the teacher for a child's slow progress. In such an instance, denial (another defense mechanism to be discussed) may be operating in conjunction with projection. In sensing that parents may be projecting blame onto her or the school, the teacher might try to help them understand that her main interest is not in *why* a child is not learning but in how to help her overcome the learning problems that have been identified. Knowledge about this mechanism can help the educator understand parent's behavior more accurately. However, some professionals resent being blamed for a parents' problems and take their remarks personally. To this, I would say that projected blame is parents' way of coping and, generally speaking, is not a conscious process designed to harm anyone.

Bibring, Dwyer, Huntington, and Vatenstein (1961) define *denial* as "literally seeing but refusing to acknowledge what one sees, or hearing and negating what is actually heard . . . " (p. 65). A more comprehensive definition of denial is that it "operates *unconsciously*, used to resolve emotional conflict and allay anxiety by disavowing thoughts, feelings, wishes needs, or external reality factors that are *consciously* intolerable" (*American Psychiatric Glossary*, 1988, p. 47; emphasis added). With regard to childhood disability, Seligman and Rosenhan (1998) assert that denial often appears when ones sense of security is threatened. For example, "the parents of a fatally ill child, much as the fatally ill themselves, often deny that anything is wrong, even though they have the diagnosis and prognosis in hand" (p. 43). With regard to childhood disability, Ross (1964) adds that "denial is one of the more primitive defenses against the threatening recognition of the discrepancy between the hoped-for healthy baby and the reality of the defective* child. Parents will try to establish the myth that there is nothing wrong with the child and since this pretense serves to protect them from anxiety, they must try to maintain the myth against great odds" (pp. 62–63). Kroth and Edge (1997) comment on denial in an educational context:

> Teachers are sometimes confronted by denying parents. When a teacher has to tell parents that their child is failing or should be referred for special testing, the parents may act as if they did not hear. They may ignore the advice, or they may go doctor shopping for another diagnosis. Although the professionals may think that time is being wasted, the denial stage is productive. It is a time that gives the parent some space to think, process, and absorb what is being presented. (p. 52)

Family members can be reinforced in denying their child's disability by professionals. Because of professionals' own anxieties against which they must defend, physicians, for example, may hedge on accurately communicating the severity of the problem, be unrealistically hopeful, or promise unattainable cures (Marshak & Seligman, 1993). Parents, aided by well-meaning but misguided professionals, secretly hold on to the belief that the problem will somehow go away or that the child will "grow out of it." Shopping around for a favorable diagnosis is caused by parent denial, which can be reinforced by professionals' inability to deal honestly with the parents. Relatedly, family members look to professionals to help them achieve a sense of pride in their child. The professionals' perceptions and communication to parents of their favorable or unfavorable sentiments toward the child affect, in part, how parents perceive their child with a disability:

> When I placed Matthew into a strange woman's arms on his first day in the infant program, I didn't know what she hoped to accomplish with my 4-week-old baby. . . . As the weeks and months passed, I

---

*"Defective," once used in the professional literature, is a term that is no longer acceptable; in fact, it is now considered to be a derogatory and repugnant reference to persons with disabilities.

sensed my baby's growing attachment to his teacher and his response
to her obvious delight whenever he accomplished a new feat. I, too,
unconsciously formed my attachment to her. . . . Professionals who
work with families in the early months of the child's life can have a
profound influence on parents. A mother may hear the first hopeful
words about her child from the teacher or therapist. And those words
and assurances can become the basis of strong attachments, acknowledged or unrealized, between parents and program staff. (in Moeller,
1986, pp. 151–152)

Gorham, DesJardins, Page, Pettis, and Scheiber (1975) pointed out
some time ago that a physician's training in the care of children with
disabilities and their parents is minimal. This gap in medical training
still exists (Darling & Peter, 1994). These authors assert that the physician, a professional, is also human and understandably uncomfortable
with the situation. They sometimes seek refuge from anxiety by pro-
nouncing a diagnosis and then terminating responsibility for and involvement with the parents, often by referring the child and parents
elsewhere. Contact with a pediatrician is often the parents' first exposure to rejection, a harsh reality to confront, especially from one perceived to be intimately involved with human problems. In their book,
Darling and Peter (1994) discuss the family–physician relationship in
some detail.

From the perspective of the child's development, denial has two
counterproductive consequences: On the one hand, parents may over-
protect their child, keeping him out of situations that would help in the
normalization process. For the parents, such exposure poses the threat
that their child's disability will become glaringly obvious to others
and, of course, heightens their awareness of the child's limitations. On
the other hand, denial may lead parents to exert tremendous pressures
for achievement on the child, leading to frustration for both child and
parents. Such pressure may lead to subsequent emotional problems
that further complicate the child's condition and impair family functioning.

It is important to recognize that what sometimes appears to be denial may in fact reflect the parents' accurate perception of their situation. Because of parents' closeness to children and opportunities to observe them, their perception of what might be contributing to their
child's problem could very well be accurate. Therefore, careful,
nondefensive listening by the teacher is essential. By the same token, if
the teacher is convinced that it is important that parents be more aware

of an aspect of their child's limitations, he might consider inviting them to visit the classroom to observe. Concerning denial, the teacher should remember the following:

> They [parents] do this, not because they are mean or unfeeling, but because they have no way of dealing with the hurt and hopelessness they feel when they think of their child. If you think the parents are rejecting their child—if they are too busy to talk about his problems or seem unconcerned about his progress—try to remember they may be unhappy people. Sometimes it is a stage parents go through when they learn of a child's disability, but if it continues, they will need more help than you can give. (Council for Exceptional Children, undated, pp. 4–5)

Rationalization, a word often used by professionals and the public, "means justification, or making a thing appear reasonable, when otherwise its irrationality would be evident. It is said that a person 'covers up,' justifies, rationalizes an act or an idea that is unreasonable and illogical" (Hensie & Campbell 1970, p. 645). Davison and Neale (1990) add that rationalization refers to "inventing a reason for an action or attitude" (p. 37). Tied into the mechanisms of denial and projection, rationalization provides an acceptable reason for an undesirable situation. For example, a parent may inform the teacher that his son is behind in his classwork because of an ill grandparent, when the evidence clearly points to a cognitive deficiency. Or in scoring significantly below what she expected on an examination, a college student may rationalize as follows: "I didn't do well on the examination because I didn't hit the sack until 2 o'clock in the morning. Also, the examination room was so hot that I had trouble concentrating." This rationalization may have a grain of truth in it. Nevertheless, one can see how it helps the individual avoid the possibility that the low examination score may reflect her lack of preparation or, even more devastating, that the material was too difficult for her to grasp.

Bibring et al. (1961) define *intellectualization* as "a systematic overdoing of thinking, deprived of its affect, in order to defend against anxiety attributable to an unacceptable impulse" (p. 68); that is, anxiety is warded off by verbal excesses, especially in situations where strong emotions are aroused. Seligman and Rosenhan (1998) add that intellectualization involves repressing the emotional aspects of an event or experience. Instead, the experience is subjected to an abstract intellectual analysis, which helps to cover up the affective aspects of an experience.

There is a distinct difference between intellectualization and being intelligent, with the former referring to a coping mechanism and the latter being an indication of one's potential. Intellectualizing parents may communicate cognitively more than with emotion, and they may tend to circumvent emotionally charged situations. To the educator, they may "come across" as more distant than other parents when they discuss their child. However, there are subtle differences in distinguishing people who intellectualize to reduce anxiety from people who have a more cognitive or analytic (some would say, a more distant) interpersonal style. One might say that an intellectualizing parent is one who has not come to terms with his child's disability. Teachers should understand this way of coping and, rather than being critical, use it to understand parents' adjustment to their child's disability.

Strong impulses, generally of an aggressive or sexual nature and considered to be unacceptable, are, at an unconscious level, deflected into socially acceptable, constructive activities. Gratification of a socially objectionable impulse in a socially valued outlet characterizes the defense mechanism of *sublimation* (Seligman & Rosenhan, 1998). For example, having the impulse to aggressively strike back at the perceived sources of a child's lack of academic or therapeutic alternatives in the community, a parent of a child with disabilities may help form a citizens group dedicated to the orderly and legal pursuit of expanded opportunities for these children. Sublimation is generally viewed as an acceptable and socially useful form of coping. For example, it is not uncommon for family members, having experienced disability in the family, to work in a human-service-related area or to become advocates for disability causes (Seligman & Darling, 1997).

Ross (1964) defines *repression* as:

> the mechanism through which unacceptable and threatening psychological content is kept from conscious awareness. Repressed activities, impulses, and conflicts which are thus excluded from consciousness are not eliminated and they continue to cause stress which may become expressed in various indirect symptoms. Because of the continuing threat posed by repressed material, other defense mechanisms are called into play, making repression the mechanism which is central to many other psychic operations. (p. 53)

Thus, repression keeps impulses and events that cause excessive anxiety essentially hidden (unconscious); yet according to psychoanalytic theory, thoughts or emotions that fall into the unconscious are manifested in some way (e.g., through denial, projection, or sublimation). Thoughts that evoke shame, guilt, humiliation, or self-deprecation are sometimes repressed. Like the other coping mechanisms, repression helps to reduce anxiety. To help alleviate the negative consequences of repressed thoughts and emotions, confronting uncomfortable parts of one's past or present by talking with an empathic counselor or psychologist can facilitate adjustment (Laborde & Seligman, 1991).

"Repression" and "suppression" are often used interchangeably, even though they are different. *Suppression* is the act of *consciously* inhibiting an impulse, idea, or emotion—a *deliberate* attempt to forget something. In talking with a parent who wishes to suppress an uncomfortable thought, one might hear something like the following: "I realize that Tommy won't ever be able to walk like other children. I find this so upsetting that I sometimes don't want to think or talk about it."

Kicking the family dog after an unnerving day at the office is the popular characterization of *displacement*, the shifting of an impulse from one source to another in order to respond to a conflict and avoid anxiety. Generally, the true object of anger or frustration is replaced by one that is more innocent and less threatening (Seligman & Rosenhan, 1998). The impulse (e.g., feeling angry and acting aggressively) does not change, but the direction of the impulse is deflected (e.g., kicking the dog instead of asserting oneself with one's boss, the real source of anger).

Deflected impulses are not always directed to an external source but are sometimes turned against oneself. Ross (1964) notes that impulses turned inward find expression through bodily symptoms, a mechanism called *somatization*. For example, after an emotionally laden meeting with the principal, a teacher may incorrectly assume the blame and responsibility for a situation that objectively is not her fault. This teacher may be particularly susceptible to guilt and self-blame, and may feel at fault for other situations not of her doing. A person may develop physical symptoms if she is guilt-ridden, often assuming self-blame when it is not warranted, and keeps these emotions hidden. Physical symptoms may include headaches, stomach problems, and the like. Some believe that more serious sequelae (such as heart disease) can result from emotions that are hidden for long periods.

A response to an uncomfortable situation, albeit generally a temporary one, is to withdraw. *Withdrawal*, a fairly common and normal reaction to a threatening situation, can become a characteristic way of responding, a signal that professional help is needed. In order to avoid a painful evaluation of their child, for example, parents may absent themselves from parent–teacher conferences. More often than not, however, parents will summon the needed courage to attend scheduled meetings, believing that no matter how uncomfortable, it is a situation that must be faced in the interest of their child. Chronic withdrawal, however, indicates that excessive anxiety may be present.

The coping mechanisms discussed here come from the psychoanalytic literature. Although psychoanalysis is not as popular as it once was, it still has its adherents in psychology, psychiatry, social work, literature, and education. In understanding families of children with disabilities, I believe that the coping or defense mechanisms described here help professionals understand behaviors that family members use to manage acute and chronic stressors. In fact, such mechanisms help us as professionals to achieve greater insights into our own reactions and behavior. However, in more recent years, other models or theories of coping have been developed, with perhaps the most cited one being that of Lazarus and Folkman (1984).

Cognitive Coping

Lazarus and Folkman theorize that coping, an interaction between the person and the environment, is dynamically and mutually reciprocal. In their model, stress is seen as a cognitive process in which the person appraises a situation for potential threats to well-being. If a situation is perceived as a threat, the person determines whether it is overtaxing his or her resources for coping. In this sense, Lazarus and Folkman's model is more cognitive and suggests a more conscious and transactional approach to dealing with stress, whereas the defense mechanisms noted earlier are more unconscious and intrapsychic (*American Psychiatric Glossary*, 1988).

According to Lazarus and Folkman (1984) coping serves two major functions, namely, to deal with the problem that is causing distress (problem-focused coping) or to regulate emotion (emotion-focused coping). In general, these authors assert that emotion-focused coping is more likely to be used when there is an appraisal that nothing (or little) can be done to change or modify a situation. In contrast, problem-focused coping strategies are designed to alter the environment or something about the person (e.g., using a new behavior to achieve a particular goal or response).

Of the different types of coping strategies that have been developed, seven types are included in either the emotion-focused or problem-focused categories. Emotion-focused coping strategies include distancing, self-control, escape–avoidance, accepting responsibility, and positive reappraisal. Problem-focused coping strategies include problem solving and confrontive coping.

An illustration of problem-focused coping is when a 56-year-old executive in an advertising firm decides to take early retirement after a heart attack. Another example is when a concert violinist develops arthritis and decides to teach the violin rather than to continue to perform.

As noted earlier, emotion-focused coping is likely to be used when people believe that they cannot change a situation and must, therefore, endure it. According to Hymovich and Hagopian (1992), emotion-focused strategies are used to "maintain hope and optimism, deny both fact and implication, or refuse to acknowledge the worst" (p. 176). An illustration of emotion-focused coping is when the father of a child with mental retardation uses distancing and escape–avoidance to deal with the anxieties aroused by his son. This would generally be a problematic solution in that as the father withdraws, the mother and other children are expected to fill the gap the father leaves. A more functional, emotion-focused strategy is positive reappraisal, where the father considers that his son is a blessing rather than a burden, and a gift worthy of love and acceptance or, alternatively, that his son has worth despite his mental retardation.

Parents of children with disabilities theoretically fall into the emotion-focused group of coping strategies due to the "unfixable" nature of their child's disability. For some parents, this assumption may be true, whereas for others, it may not (Houser & Seligman, 1991). Some parents unconditionally accept their child, reinterpreting the child as one who requires love, support, and little else. However, other parents assertively react to childhood disability by mobilizing the family's resources to help their child walk, talk, become integrated into the community, and eventually become semi-independent. These parents summon available social support to help them achieve these goals. Thus, it is certainly possible for parents, facing a relatively unchangeable situation, to engage in problem-focused coping strategies.

A final system of coping—one that bears some resemblance to the Lazarus and Folkman model—supports the use of the following coping styles:

- Passive appraisal (ignoring a problem in the hope it will go away)
- Reframing (changing the way one thinks about a problem in order to solve it and/or to make it seem less stressful)
- Spiritual support (deriving comfort and guidance from one's spiritual beliefs)

- Social support (receiving practical and emotional assistance from friends and family)
- Professional support (receiving assistance from professionals and human service agencies) (Olson et al., 1984)

The purpose of this section is to advise the reader about common coping mechanisms or styles that help teachers assess how parents choose to negotiate life with their child who has a disability. Teachers need to understand that coping mechanisms help not only family members but also professionals deal with difficult and anxiety-provoking situations in their personal and professional lives. They are common reactions to life stressors and are not to be interpreted as unusual or peculiar responses. Furthermore, in the disability area, the adoption of any particular coping style is a function of numerous factors, such as the family of origin, style of coping, the severity of a child's disability, the stigma attributed to the disability, the availability of support services, and the like.

RELATED CONCEPTS

In addition to the basic family systems models and coping methods discussed earlier, several other concepts are germane to the understanding of family functioning.

The Social Ecology Point of View

In the early writing on families with a member who is disabled, researchers defined the unit of study or intervention in very narrow terms, focusing primarily on the family member with the disability and ignoring the family as a legitimate focus. In the field of childhood disability, the first "family" studies focused on the interaction between the mother and her child. Later, siblings, fathers, and grandparents were included as family members who were affected by disability and who could also affect the person with a disability. The consideration of the family as a dynamic, interdependent unit was a profound step, yet even these broader views of family life were too narrow. We know that persons with disabilities do not live in isolation—they typically reside within a family context. Similarly, the family lives in a broader social context. The conceptualization of the family within a social ecology framework has been discussed extensively by Bronfenbrenner (1979) and has always been the focus of sociologists concerned with the family (Seligman & Darling, 1997).

Similar to boundary concerns between subsystems in the family systems model, the social ecology model is also concerned with the permeability of the family when it interacts with environmental systems, for example, whether a family with a member who is disabled is open to the supportive influences of other, similarly situated families (e.g., support groups) or amenable to the educational system and to assistance from social service agencies or other sources of help. The permeability of the family vis-à-vis the environment may influence the amount of isolation, support, and stress it experiences. Contrast, for example, family members who cooperatively work with their child's teacher, the medical community, or the social service system, get involved in support groups with other families, and utilize available respite care services with family members who feel that they should "take care of their own," resist medical advice, view their child's education with suspicion, isolate themselves from others in similar circumstances, and refuse social services. Possibly due to the family's personal philosophy, determined by the family of origin and religious and cultural values, the second family will not feel supported and connected to others, and will be suspicious of offers of help. By the same token, some families have rich resources within the nuclear and extended family that allow them to cope with minimal outside support.

The social ecology point of view asserts that a family can be affected by remote events. For example, political and economic factors bear a direct relationship to the funds available for educational and social services for persons with disabilities. An international conflict can mobilize sentiment that supports arms buildup and not educational and social services. Thus, the dynamics of the family members can be influenced by a variety of external and remote events. In light of this reality, a broad conceptualization of the forces that impinge on family life provides additional meaning to understanding the family.

Bronfenbrenner's (1979) social ecology model includes the microsystems, mesosystem, ecosystem, and macrosystem, with each system reflecting activity increasingly removed from the family but nevertheless influencing it. This model is easily applied to families with children who are disabled.

The *microsystem* constitutes the pattern of activities, roles, and interpersonal relations experienced within the family. In it, one finds the following components: mother–father, mother–disabled child, mother–nondisabled child, father–nondisabled child, disabled child–

nondisabled child. This pattern of subsystems resembles the family systems theory already discussed.

The microsystem functions in a *mesosystem* comprising a wide range of settings in which a family actively participates. The following combine to make up the mesosystem: medical and health care workers, teachers, the extended family, friends and neighbors, work associates, other parents, and other local community factors.

In the *ecosystem*, settings in which the family is not actively involved can impact the family, such as the mass media, health care systems, social welfare agencies, and educational systems.

And, finally, there is the *macrosystem*, an ideological or belief system inherent in the social institutions of society, which includes ethnic/cultural, religious, socioeconomic, and political elements.

In understanding families, it is not sufficient to study only certain family members. It is becoming increasingly incumbent to examine the family within the context of larger social, economic, and political realities.

Stress

One of the emotional consequences of living in a fast-moving world is stress. A contributing factor to stress is the adjustment required as major changes take place in the family (e.g., a child leaves home to attend college, the birth of a newborn, or death of a grandparent). Contributing to these factors is the added stress inherent in coping with a chronic illness or disability. Stressors can be defined as either expected or unexpected events (Gladding, 1998). Expected stressors include such things as financial problems, attempting to cope with children's behavior, and insufficient couple or personal time. Unexpected stressors are not predictable. "Some family-life situations take family members by surprise or are beyond their control. If life events come too soon, are delayed, or fail to materialize, the health, happiness, and well-being of all involved may be affected" (p. 39).

Generally speaking, living and stress go hand in hand. According to a popular saying, "If you ain't got stress, you ain't living." Yet excessive and unrelenting stress can take its toll on one's emotional and physical well-being. Chronic illness or disability tend to be time-extended stressors.

Hill (1949) developed a model of stress, often cited in the family literature (McCubbin & Patterson, 1983; Wikler, 1981), called the ABCX Family Crisis Model where *A* (the stressor event) interacts with B (the family's crisis meeting resources), which interacts with C (the definition the family makes of the event) to produce X (the crisis).

The stressor (the A factor) is a life event or transition that produces change in the family system. The family's goals, boundaries, patterns of interaction, roles, or values may be threatened by change caused by a stressor (McCubbin & Patterson, 1983). A stressor event, for example, may be the family's need to increase its income due to the financial problems a disability has caused. The added factor of disability in the family can place demands on the roles and functions of family members, alter their collective and individual goals, and affect the family's interaction.

Family resources (the B factor) represents the family's ability to prevent an event or change in the family from causing a crisis (McCubbin & Patterson, 1983). The B factor is the family's capacity to meet obstacles and shift its course of action. This factor relates directly to the notion that the family's flexibility and quality of relationship *prior* to the disability may be an important predictor of its ability to cope. For example, a cohesive family that has a generally positive outlook and extended family support, both psychologically and instrumentally, can appropriately utilize community resources to cope successfully with childhood disability.

The C factor is how the family defines the seriousness of the stressor. This factor also reflects the family's values and previous experience in dealing with change and meeting crises. The B and C factors probably account for most of the positive coping skills we see families exhibit. The C factor is particularly useful for professionals in their efforts to intervene. A family's appraisal of its situation may be bleak, thrusting family members into a state of depression and anomie. The professional can help by invoking more positive appraisals of the child by helping family members refocus. For example, by speaking about what the child with the disability *can do* to contribute to and enrich family life, educators can help to give new and more positive meaning to the family's situation.

Collectively, the three factors influence the family's ability to prevent the stressor event from creating a crisis (the X factor), which reflects the family's inability to restore balance and stability. However, stress may never become a crisis if the family is able to use existing resources and define the situation as a manageable event.

The next section explores various resources and interactions that can help families cope with disability.

RESOURCES

Patterson (1988) identified three categories of resources for families: personal resources, family systems resources, and community resources.

Personal Resources

Personal resources entail individual personality characteristics derived primarily from social interaction. For example, self-esteem is a pervasive human characteristic that mediates one's response to life events and contributes to a sense of mastery and self-efficacy. Patterson (1988) cited studies suggesting that high self-esteem is associated with better adherence to treatment regimens and that diabetic children with a positive self-concept evidence better control of their diabetes. Also, high parental self-esteem was noted as contributing to the well-being of a chronically ill child. In families with a diabetic child, parental self-esteem was a key factor in predicting better functioning and child self-esteem (Patterson, 1988).

Educators can contribute to the self-esteem of a child with a disability by focusing on strengths and by treating the child with dignity and respect. As mentioned earlier, in working with the family, focusing on a person's abilities can help increase feelings of efficacy, control, and worthiness. Particularly important is the underlying prizing attitude conveyed by the teacher to the family and to the family member with a disability. Uncaring attitudes lower a person's self-esteem. As noted earlier, family members look to professionals to confirm their healthy view of themselves and their child. When it is not forthcoming, people suffer a loss of self-esteem. Professionals must not contribute negatively to stressful family situations that challenge a person's sense of dignity, worthiness, and efficacy. Some years ago, Ross (1964) expressed his beliefs regarding professionals who work with families:

> No amount of exhortation can make a rejecting person accepting, a frigid person warm, or a narrow-minded person understanding. Those charged with the selection, education, and training of new members of the helping professions will need to keep in mind that the presence of certain personality characteristics makes the difference between a truly helpful professional and one who leaves a trace of misery and confusion in the wake of his activities. (pp. 75–76)

Some professionals' behaviors that contribute to negative self-evaluation and negative attitudes toward professionals include abruptness, inattentiveness, misinformation or lack of information, and an attitude of coldness or aloofness. Family members are puzzled by inept, inaccurate, and ill-timed professional advice, and by the communication of information in professional jargon. Education professionals who engage in this type of behavior need to understand the impact their attitudes and behavior can have on family members.

Family System Resources

Patterson (1988) cites numerous studies in support of the claim that the family can supply many of the resources needed to cope with disability. In particular, family organization seems to be a crucial variable and includes such elements as clarity of rules and expectations, family routines, and clear role allocation. Clear generational boundaries, with a parental hierarchy that cooperatively works to make decisions and establish and maintain child discipline, are also essential organizational attributes.

In the case of parental disability, a parental hierarchy concerned with decisions and discipline may be undermined, but it should not, because parental disability should not rob people of taking roles that they are capable of assuming. Parents feel pride in their nurturing and guidance functions, and children feel secure in a warm, caring family that is directed by parents. Therefore, fathers and mothers should make every effort to continue their parenting in spite of a disability. In some instances, however, some children may be pressed into parental (caretaking) roles that they may not be prepared to assume when family disability strikes.

Due to changes in circumstances and needs, the family organization needs to be sufficiently flexible to meet these changes. With regard to childhood disabilities, a child's condition may worsen, improve, or remain the same (Rolland, 1993). Family flexibility is important whether the change is positive or negative. In conditions that are cyclical in nature (e.g., in multiple sclerosis), family members may need to change their roles depending on whether the condition allows for a full range of activities, whether there are some restrictions, and whether hospitalization is required.

Other family resources include an active family recreation orientation in which an atmosphere of normalcy is maintained and cohesion increases as the family learns to cope with the demands of the disability (Patterson, 1988; Wallinga, Paquio, & Skeen, 1987). In the case of childhood disability, the father's support helps to set the tone for the family (Lamb & Meyer, 1991). As discussed in more detail later, the father's acceptance or rejection of the disability appears to affect the experience of other family members, and his psychological and instrumental support helps to lessen the family's burden.

As noted earlier, family members are resources for each other when they can achieve a balance in their interactions between being too·close (enmeshed) or too distant. Family members, when too close, are overly reactive to each other and suffocate attempts at independence. They do not provide the kind of emotional support that results in security and self-efficacy.

Marital relationships characterized by mutual support, intimacy, and shared goals are an important resource in effective family functioning (Patterson, 1988). When childhood disability occurs, it is essential for family members to maintain a balanced life by finding time for themselves. Respite from caretaking by pursuing hobbies and other personal or collective interests provides balance for family members who must devote considerable energy to help manage and support the family member who has a disability. Teachers who see parents as overly involved with their child to the exclusion of all pleasures can suggest to them that they develop or resume activities that enhance their growth or pleasure. Often, such a suggestion helps to facilitate a happier lifestyle for both parents, the child with a disability, and the other children in the family. This type of communication from the teacher should be timed properly, after a good relationship has been established. It might come after parents have discussed the overwhelming nature of the child's demands and burden of the stress they feel with the teacher. For example, the teacher might say:

> "It sounds as if you're experiencing considerable stress lately. I'm sure this situation concerns you, and you may not be sure how to make the situation better. I'm not a psychologist or counselor, but I've read and heard that some families with children who have disabilities sort of reevaluate their circumstances and consider making some changes in the family to help lessen stress. There are times when families need to balance their lives by developing new interests or activities, or consider going back to some old hobbies. I'm not sure if this makes sense in your situation but I thought I'd mention this to you. What do you think?"

Some parents may experience guilt in pursuing personal interests and goals. They may see this as selfish and egotistical. Professionals can give family members "permission" by noting how such activities can increase satisfying family relationships.

Finally, a communication style that encourages the expression of emotions is particularly adaptive for families that experience conflicting and powerful emotions. In the long run, the expression of emotions deepens relationships and prevents smoldering emotions from building and causing harm to the family.

Community Resources

The final type of help for families is community resources (Patterson, 1988). Although not really a community resource per se, the extended family can provide emotional and practical help (Seligman, 1991b). For example, in childhood disability, grandparents have provided help by babysitting, shopping for the family, taking the child for medical appointments, helping with domestic chores, and even by helping financially (Seligman, 1991b). Another resource for families is respite care (Upshur, 1991). By having a trained respite care worker remain with the family member who is disabled, other members can go shopping, enjoy dinner out or a movie, and, in some instances, take a vacation. Most communities now have respite care services available to which educators can direct families burdened by excessive caretaking demands. We know that families are better able to cope when financial resources such as supplemental security income (SSI) are available. Enabling legislation helps to establish programs and policies that improve the lives of persons with disabilities (e.g., the Americans with Disabilities Act).

Another source of community support is from others who are coping with the same or a similar disability, namely, peer self-help or support groups (Lieberman, 1990). Support groups represent a powerful medium of emotional support and practical help. The quick identification of persons in similar circumstances helps family members feel less alone in their struggles and provides a network of friends who understand and can provide instrumental assistance (Seligman, 1993). Here, again, teachers can direct families to appropriate support groups in the community. Feeling isolated, alone, and unsupported is a particularly vexing problem for families of children who have rare disorders. Families with children who have Down syndrome or physical disabilities typically know other families who are coping with a child who has a similar exceptionality. Children suffering from rare disorders are generally severely disabled. Families of children with rare disorders have fewer interpersonal or social resources, yet have frequent contact with the numerous professionals that provide services for their child.

AN INTRODUCTION TO FAMILY
AND SOCIAL SYSTEMS

Before we examine how families respond to childhood disability in Chapter 4, it is useful to consider family and social systems concepts. These concepts form the backdrop against which we can examine family reactions to disability. Without a basic understanding of systems concepts, our ability to grasp the meaning of childhood disability within the family is limited.

Only in recent years have family systems concepts been taken seriously by professionals who work with families with a chronically disabled member. As we know, a major drawback of the singular focus on the individual who has a disability is the omission of other family members. In some instances, nondisabled family members (e.g., siblings) may cope poorly (Fanos, 1996; McHugh, 1999). The concentrated focus on the disabled family member is also short-sighted in that it neglects the dynamic nature of family functioning. As noted earlier, disability that affects one family member in turn affects the entire system.

The reluctance to embrace a broader, or ecological, perspective may have been partially caused by theories that focus on intrapsychic rather than interpersonal processes. Related to this is psychoanalytic theory's almost exclusive focus on the mother, with a particular focus on the mother–child relationship. Parke (1981) notes that fathers, for example, are ignored purposely because of the assumption that they are less important than mothers in influencing the developing child. Extant theories reflect the traditional conception of the remote father. Bowlby (1951) also stresses that mothers are the first and most important object of infant attachment and that fathers play only a supporting role. As we will see later, contemporary views hold that fathers can, and perhaps should, share a central role in the family with the mother.

Presently, there is considerable interest in integrating family systems theories with the available information about children, adolescents, and adults with disabilities and their families (see, e.g., Blacher, 1984; Turk & Kerns, 1985; Turnbull & Turnbull, 1986; Imber-Black, 1988; Seligman, 1991a; Seligman & Darling, 1997; Darling & Peter, 1994; Hornby, 1994; Marshak, Seligman, & Prezant, 1999).

The purpose of this section is to provide a conceptual lens for understanding family functioning in general. The next chapter more specifically deals with family functioning when a child with a disability is a part of the family unit.

FAMILY SYSTEMS THEORY

Some years ago, Minuchin (1974) captured the essence of the interactive nature of the family:

> The individual influences his context and is influenced by it in constantly recurring sequences of interaction. The individual who lives within a family is a member of a social system to which he must adapt. His actions are governed by the characteristics of the system and these characteristics include the effects of his own past actions. The individual responds to stresses in other parts of the system to which he adapts; and he may contribute significantly to stressing other members of the system. The individual can be approached as a subsystem, or part of the system, but the whole must be taken into account. (p. 9)

As noted at the beginning of this chapter and repeated here because it is such a central concept, the family operates as an interactive unit; what affects one member affects all members. von Bertalanffy (1968) observed that all living systems are composed of interdependent parts and that the interaction of these parts creates characteristics not contained in the separate entities; thus, as noted by Carter and McGoldrick (1980), the family is more than the sum of its parts. Therefore, family life can best be understood by studying the relationship among its members.

However, before one can grasp the dynamic nature of family functioning, it is imperative to have an understanding of the characteristics, both static and dynamic, that comprise most family units. We turn, then, to Turnbull, Summers, and Brotherson's (1984) and Turnbull and Turnbull's (1986) conceptualization of the family. These authors have made a noteworthy effort to apply family systems theory to the study of families of children with disabilities.

FAMILY STRUCTURE

Family structure speaks to the variety of characteristics that serve to make families unique, including membership characteristics, cultural factors, and ideological style.

Membership Characteristics

As Turnbull and colleagues (1984) note, much of the literature on families with disabled members is based on the assumption of family homogeneity. Families differ with regard to numerous membership characteristics. Some of the differences include extended family members who may or may not reside in the household; single-parent families; families with an unemployed breadwinner; or families in which there is a major psychological disorder, such as substance abuse, mental illness, or the continuing influence on the family of a deceased family member. Membership characteristics change over time (Rolland, 1993). For example, families experience the so-called "empty nest" syndrome after the youngest child leaves home. When that happens, the adults who are left must negotiate new communication and relationship patterns.

Cultural Factors

Cultural beliefs are one of the most static components of the family and can play an important role in shaping its ideological style, interactional patterns, and functional priorities (Turnbull et al., 1984; McGoldrick et al., 1996). Cultural style may be influenced by ethnic, racial, or religious factors, or by socioeconomic status. In her review of the literature, Schorr-Ribera (1987) points out that culturally based beliefs affect the manner in which families adapt to a child with a disability and can also influence their usage of and level of trust in caregiver and caregiving institutions. The effect of cultural and ethnic factors on family beliefs and behavior has received increased attention in recent years (Seligman & Darling, 1997; Harry, 1992; McGoldrick et al., 1996). As noted earlier in this chapter, when considering cultural differences, we must be aware of the influence of social class and poverty—characteristics that cut across racial and ethnic lines. Furthermore, there are differences within cultures, making it dangerous to paint all people from a particular group with the same brush. For example, the Hispanic population in the United States is not a homogeneous group but derives its heterogeneity from religious and secular values, and beliefs according to the country of origin (e.g., Mexico, Cuba, Puerto Rico). Finally, there are religious and regional differences among other cultural entities that must be considered before making any declarations about the characteristics of people from a particular cultural group (Seligman & Darling, 1997).

Ideological Style

Ideological style is based on a family's beliefs, values, and coping behaviors, and is also influenced by subcultural beliefs (McGoldrick et al., 1996). For example, Jewish families place a great deal of importance on intellectual achievement. Such academic achievement may be sought in part to enable Jews to pursue professional opportunities designed to help them escape the repercussions of discrimination; therefore, they strongly urge their children to attend college. A college degree is seen as a means toward achieving independence/autonomy. Italian families, which tend to emphasize family closeness and affection, may view college attendance as a threat to family cohesiveness. This may be more a factor in families from the "old country" than in American-born Italians, attesting again to the diversity of various cultural groups. Other beliefs and values may be handed down from generation to generation and influence how family members interact with one another and with other families and other systems (such as schools and government agencies).

While a family's response to childhood disability may be influenced by ideological style, the reverse may also be true, namely, that such a child may influence a family's values. For example, when a child is born with a disability, a family not only responds to the event itself but must also confront its beliefs about people who have disabilities. Since chronic illness or disability does not discriminate on racial, cultural, socioeconomic, or value-based grounds, a child with a disability may be born to a family that is very dogmatic and prejudiced. In such an instance, the family must grapple with what the child means to them psychologically and practically (Brinthaupt, 1991). In addition, family members must also examine their beliefs about persons with minority-group status, namely, persons with disabilities. The birth of a child with a disability thus results in a double shock to the family. In addition, there is little doubt that this circumstance has the potential to create life-altering changes in family members. It can change the trajectory of life goals, accomplishments, and occupations.

Only the phenomenological experience of individual family members determines whether life trajectories are positive or negative.

Ideological style influences the coping mechanisms of families. Coping was defined earlier as any response designed to reduce stress. Coping behaviors can motivate the family either to change the situation or to change the perceived meaning of the situation.

Family Interaction

We have established that it is important for professionals to realize that children with disabilities do not function in isolation. This reaffirms the notion that persons live within a context—the family—and that when something happens to one member of the family, everyone is affected.

To say that a family is a unit comprised of a certain number of individuals and that they function in a dynamic interrelationship provides only a partial picture of how a family operates. Turnbull and colleagues (1984) elaborate on the four components of the interactional system: subsystems, cohesion, adaptability, and communication.

Subsystems

Within a family there are the following four subsystems:

1. Marital: husband and wife.
2. Parental: parent and child.
3. Sibling: child and child.
4. Extrafamilial: extended family, friends, professionals, and so forth.

The makeup of subsystems is affected by the structural characteristics of families (e.g., size of extrafamilial network, single mother or father, number of children) and by the current life-cycle stage (the family life cycle is discussed later).

Professionals need to be cautious when they intervene in a subsystem. For example, an intervention designed to strengthen the bond between a mother and her child can have implications for the mother's relationship with her husband and other children. The family needs to be considered within the context of the other subsystems, so that the resolution of one problem does not bring about the emergence of others. Perhaps such difficulties can be minimized by including (rather than excluding) family members. Unfortunately, in parent conferences, fathers are often absent from the marital subsystem. For some families, father-absent conferences can be problematic; therefore, the educator is encouraged to have both parents present during parent conferences.

Cohesion and Adaptability

Subsystems describe *who* in the family will interact, whereas cohesion and adaptability describe *how* family members interact.

Cohesion can best be characterized by the concepts of enmeshment and disengagement. Highly enmeshed families have weak boundaries between subsystems and can be characterized as over-involved and overprotective (Minuchin, 1974). Such families have difficulty allowing for a sense of individuality. Overprotective families can have deleterious effects on their children with disabilities. Such families experience considerable anxiety in "letting go" of their children and hence may keep them from participating in growth-promoting activities that encourage independence and positive self-esteem.

Conversely, disengaged families have rigid subsystem boundaries (Minuchin, 1974). With regard to a family with a child who has a disability, interactions may be characterized by underinvolvement. Turnbull and Turnbull (1986) describe two situations that illustrate disengagement: one in which a father denies the disability and withdraws from both marital and parental interactions, and the other in which grandparents reject the child with a disability to the point of not allowing the child to join the family during holiday meals, thus creating considerable tension in the family.

Well-functioning families are characterized by a balance between enmeshment and disengagement (Gladding, 1998). Boundaries between subsystems are clearly defined, and family members feel both a close bond and a sense of autonomy. Enmeshment and disengagement, then, represent the outer boundaries of a continuum; in the approximate middle of the continuum one finds well-functioning families.

Adaptability refers to the family's ability to change in response to a stressful situation (Olson, Russell, & Sprenkle, 1980). Rigid families do not change in response to stress, and chaotic families are characterized by instability and inconsistent change. A rigid family has difficulty adjusting to the demands of caring for a significantly impaired child. The father's rigid breadwinner role, for example, does not allow him to help with domestic chores or to assist with child care ("woman's work"), thereby placing an inordinate burden on the mother; thus, the mother must put all of her energies into caretaking responsibilities that leave little time for the other children in the family or for interacting with other people. This family is in jeopardy of becoming isolated and dysfunctional.

A chaotic family has few rules to live by, and those that do exist are often changed. There is no family leader, and there may be endless negotiations and frequent role changes (Turnbull & Turnbull, 1986). Chaotic families seem to move frequently from a sense of closeness or enmeshment to one of distance and hostility–disengagement. When change occurs, families who interact in a functional way maintain a balance between emotional unity and autonomy, between reacting to change and a sense of stability, and between closed and random communication (Turnbull & Turnbull, 1986).

Communication

From a family systems perspective, communications breakdowns reflect a problematic system rather than faulty people. Communications problems reside in the interactions between people, not within people (Turnbull & Turnbull, 1986). When professionals work with families from a systems point of view, the emphasis is on changing patterns of interaction and not on changing individuals. They avoid placing blame on one family member or another and instead attempt to explore the factors that contribute to problematic communication patterns. Family members sometimes believe that a particular member is responsible for the problems they are experiencing, but they usually discover that difficulties often reside in faulty communications, not faulty people.

Family Functions

Family functions are products, or outputs, of family interaction (Turnbull et al., 1984). They reflect the *results* of interaction in terms of the ability to meet the needs of the family's members. To carry out functions successfully requires considerable interdependence between the family and its extrafamilial network. Also, families differ in regard to the priorities they attach to different functions and to who is expected to carry out certain functions.

The following reflect typical family functions:

1. economic (e.g., generating income, paying bills);
2. domestic/health care (e.g., transportation, purchasing and preparing food, medical visits);
3. recreation (e.g., hobbies, recreation for the family and for the individual);
4. socialization (e.g., developing social skills, interpersonal relationships);
5. self-identity (e.g., recognizing strengths and weaknesses, sense of belonging);
6. affection (e.g., intimacy, nurturing);
7. educational/vocational (e.g., career choice, development of work ethic, homework). (Turnbull & Turnbull, 1986, p. 80)

A child with a disability residing with the family, especially a severely impaired child, can increase consumptive demands without proportionately increasing the family's productive capability (Turnbull et al., 1984); that is, a family must spend more of its energies and available time to attend to issues related to the disability or illness and have less time for leisure, recreational, educational, social, and career issues. As a result, a child with a disability residing in the least restrictive environment, namely, the family, may unintentionally generate a restrictive environment for all family members.

Furthermore, it is conceivable that the child can change the family's self-identity, reduce its earning capacity, constrict its recreational and social opportunities, and affect career decisions. One can see in fairly concrete terms how disability or chronic illness can affect the family by reflecting on the family functions noted earlier. For example, the family's economic, health care, and caretaking tasks leave few resources for other family functions. This discussion also puts into perspective the notion that well-functioning families need to be flexible and open to change.

The discussion thus far has focused on potential family problems. It is just as conceivable that children with disabilities can have a positive effect on family functions (Featherstone, 1980; Grossman, 1972; Turnbull et al., 1993; Turnbull et al., 1995). For example, in one study, Turnbull, Brotherson, and Summers (1985) reported that families perceive a major positive contribution of a retarded member to be related to guidance, affection, and self-definition. In this study, parents and siblings describe positive attitudinal and value changes that they attribute to the retarded family member. In Turnbull and Turnbull's (1985) book, *Parents Speak Out*, Turnbull et al.'s (1993) *Cognitive Coping, Families, and Disability*, and Trainer's (1991) *Differences in Common*, contributors identify numerous positive benefits a child with a disability can have on families.

Some authors question the emphasis placed on the role of parents as teachers of their child (Seligman, 1979; Turnbull et al., 1984). Parents have many roles to play; the role of adjunct educator is only one of several functions. Professionals need to be concerned about how the overburdening of one role affects the others. Also, in asking parents to assume an educational function, it is useful to inquire about the parents' wish to take on that role and whether they are comfortable with it or feel prepared to assume it. Families are sometimes asked to do more at home with their child than the family system can tolerate. As noted elsewhere, too much stress can be placed on the family when professionals fail to coordinate the activities that family members assume.

With certain types of childhood impairments, a family may be given "homework" by the child's teacher, speech therapist, and physical therapist, among others. There needs to be some monitoring of the functions professionals ask a family to assume and a recognition of how overburdening one family function can affect the successful performance of others. Professionals belonging to various medical, social, and educational systems can help alleviate stress, but they can also contribute to it; therefore, professionals "must appreciate the requirement for ongoing interaction with larger systems, the stress generated thereby, and the need to intervene in ways that promote autonomy, enhance family resources, and facilitate empowerment of the family on behalf of their handicapped member" (Imber-Black, 1988, p. 105).

FAMILY LIFE CYCLE

The family life cycle is a series of developmental stages. During a particular stage, the family's lifestyle is relatively stable, and each member is engaged in developmental tasks related to that period of life (Duvall, 1957; Gladding, 1998). For example, a family with two late-adolescent children is coping with the usual intensity and ambivalence of adolescent life in addition to the concerns that characterize adult (the parents') midlife. Change occurs for this family when one of the children leaves home (e.g., to attend college), which affects the family structure (i.e., a reduction from four to three persons at home) and may affect other aspects of family life, such as family interaction and communication. These life-cycle stages are predictable and, therefore, anticipated by family members. In contrast, childhood disability is not anticipated and may be an "out-of-phase" or "off time" event. An illustration of an "off time" event is when a child becomes disabled and necessarily dependent on the family at age 18 as a result of a car accident. For most families, this is a time when children begin "launching" and separating from their parents, not becoming more dependent on them. Nonnormal or "out-of-phase" occurrences create greater problems and, therefore, greater stress than predictable, "on time" events (Rolland, 1993).

Six to 24 developmental stages have been identified (Carter & McGoldrick, 1980). Olson and colleagues (1984) identify seven stages, which are discussed here and include coupling, childbearing, school age, adolescence, launching, postparenting, and aging.

Each stage has its own developmental tasks; for example, parenting is important during the childbearing stage and less crucial during the postparental stage. Such functions are highly age related; for example, physical care by parents is essential during infancy, and educational and vocational guidance are important when children are in high school and college. Whereas bonding and attachment are vital in infancy, letting go is important when children reach late adolescence. Thus, a key aspect of life-cycle stages is the change in function required of families over time.

Developmental transitions (moving from one stage to another) can be a major source of stress and possibly even family dysfunction. According to a study by Olson and colleagues (1984), "launching" creates the greatest amount of family stress. However, in families where "launching" may not be possible due to chronic disability, stress may be present, as the family members are frustrated by their inability to "move on."

Turnbull and Turnbull (1986) relate the development stages derived from systems theorists to the stress experienced by families with children who have disabilities. Below, for each pertinent stage identified by Olson and colleagues (1984), are listed some illustrative stress factors:

1. Childbearing: Getting an accurate diagnosis; making emotional adjustments; informing other family members.
2. School age: Clarifying personal views regarding mainstreaming versus segregated placements; dealing with reactions of the child's peer group; arranging for child care and extracurricular activities.

3. Adolescence: Adjusting for chronicity of the child's disability; dealing with issues of sexuality; coping with peer isolation and rejection; planning for the child's vocational future.
4. Launching: Recognizing and adjusting to the family's continuing responsibility; deciding on appropriate residential placement; dealing with the lack of socialization opportunities for the disabled family member.
5. Postparenting: Reestablishing relationship with spouse (i.e., if child has been successfully launched); interacting with the disabled member's residential service providers.

This chapter has explored family systems concepts. These concepts pertain to all families as they move through the family life cycle. As noted, family life-cycle theory proposes that different behaviors and experiences characterize different life-cycle stages. Roles that are appropriate and helpful for one stage may be inappropriate and nonfunctional in another situation. The other key theoretical notion is that as inevitable change occurs in one part of the family, all other parts are also in some way affected. This chapter also acknowledged the role of stress in families and how personal, family, and social resources can ameliorate the effects of chronic stress. Chapter 4 concentrates more specifically on family response to childhood disability/illness.

4

Family Reaction
to Childhood Disability

T here are two major theories that pertain to how family members respond to the birth of an infant with a disability. Stage theory holds that family members negotiate a series of states/phases that begins with shock/disbelief and culminates in acceptance. The other prominent theory suggests that parents experience lifelong sadness or chronic sorrow. A third theory suggests that some families experience a combination of the two. The chapter begins with a discussion of stage theory, often referred to as the stages of mourning.

STAGES OF MOURNING

Since the birth of a child with a disability is experienced as a traumatic and life-altering event, there has been considerable interest in the initial and subsequent responses of family members to this occurrence (Rolland, 1993; Seligman & Darling, 1997; Marsh, 1993; Marshak et al., 1999). In light of this, there have been a number of efforts to chart the phases/stages parents experience after they have been informed of their child's disability. Blacher (1984) lists 24 studies that present some variant of stage theory. However, before exploring these reactions to the birth of a child with a disability, it is essential to acknowledge that prior to childbirth, parents have limited experience with disability. As noted in Chapter 1, however, they may have been exposed to common stereotypes and stigmatizing attitudes toward persons with disabilities that pervade our culture. As a result, during the prenatal period, most parents dread the possibility of giving birth to a child with a disability. As one mother of a Down syndrome child said, "I remember thinking, before I got married, it would be the worst thing that could ever happen to me" (Darling, 1979, p. 124). Parents' concerns are heightened when they know of other families who have children with disabilities.

Some parents claim to have had premonitions that something was wrong with their baby (Seligman & Darling, 1997). Their concerns seem to have been based on personal experience, as their expectations of what pregnancy should be like did not fit their actual experience of pregnancy. Childbirth classes prepare parents to expect a normal child, so that when an infant with a disability is born, they are not prepared for the shock. However, with the advent of modern technology, some childhood disabilities are being diagnosed prenatally. In cases of prenatal diagnosis, anticipatory grieving may be tempered by the hope that a misdiagnosis has occurred.

The following stages noted have been used in reference to families of children with special needs in response to the observation that the birth of an infant with disabilities is a traumatic loss that is often experienced by the parents as the death of the expected normal, healthy child (Solnit & Stark, 1961).

Duncan (1977) adapted Kübler-Ross's (1969) stages that characterize reactions to impending death. The stages should be viewed flexibly due to the complexity of the adjustment process and because of the variability of individual responses. The stages are as follows:

1. Shock/denial
2. Bargaining
3. Anger
4. Depression

Shock and *denial* are the parents' initial response. Denial appears to operate on an unconscious level to ward off unbearable anxiety in the face of a life-altering event. It can serve a useful, buffering purpose early on, but denial can cause difficulties if it persists. If, over time and in the face of clear evidence, parents continue to deny the existence of their child's disability, the professional needs to be cautious that

- Children are not pushed beyond their capabilities;
- Parents do not make endless and pointless visits to professionals to get an acceptable diagnosis;
- Parents do not fail to utilize social services designed to help them cope and to help the child achieve attainable levels of potential.

During this stage, parents report feeling confusion, numbness, disorganization, and helplessness. Some parents are unable to hear much of what they are told when the child's diagnosis is communicated to them.

> One mother told me that when the pediatrician told her that her 18-month-old son had cerebral palsy she "burst into tears" and didn't hear anything else. Another mother recalled how she had listened very calmly as the neurologist explained the extent of the brain damage her 14-year-old daughter had sustained as the result of a car accident. Then she got in her car and began to drive home, but after a few hundred yards, as she was crossing a bridge, she felt sick and her legs felt like they'd turned to jelly, so she got out of the car and leaned over the side of the bridge to get some air. (Hornby, 1994, p. 16)

It is important for professionals to realize that after communicating a diagnosis, parents may not be in an emotional state to hear about the details of the disability. Explanations about etiology, course, and prognosis may fall on deaf ears, often necessitating a follow-up interview. Professionals (physicians for the most part) need to deliver the diagnosis honestly and with compassion, and respond to any questions the parents may have.

The *bargaining* phase is characterized by a type of magical or fantasy thinking. The underlying theme is that if the parent works extra hard, the child will improve. A child's improved condition is compensation for hard work, being useful to others, or contributing to a worthy cause. For example, during bargaining, parents may join local groups in activities that benefit a particular cause. Another manifestation of the bargaining phase is that parents may turn to religion or look for a miracle.

As parents realize that their child will not improve significantly, *anger* develops. There may be anger at God ("Why me?") or at oneself or one's spouse for having produced the child or for not helping. Anger is frequently projected onto professionals for not healing the child (doctors) or for not helping their child make significant learning gains (teachers). Anger can be related to an unsympathetic community, insensitive professionals, inadequate services, fatigue due to long hospital stays, and the like. Also, excessive guilt can turn anger inward, so that a parent (particularly the mother) blames herself for the disability.

Expressing anger is often cathartic and cleansing, and it can reduce the negative effect of powerful emotions, but when parents realize that their anger does not change their child's condition, and when they accept the chronic nature of the disability and its implications for the family, *depression* may set in. For many parents, depression (or having the "blues") is temporary or episodic, and it is generally considered a normal reaction to a traumatic event.

Hornby (1994) believes that *detachment* sometimes follows anger. Parents report feeling empty and that nothing seems to matter. Life has lost its meaning. This reaction is thought to indicate that the parent is reluctantly beginning to accept the reality of the disability. This, then, is a turning point in the adaptation process.

Acceptance is achieved when parents demonstrate some of the following characteristics:

1. They are able to discuss their child's shortcomings with relative ease.
2. They evidence a balance between encouraging independence and showing love.
3. They are able to collaborate with professionals to make realistic short- and long-term plans.
4. They pursue personal interests unrelated to their child.
5. They can discipline appropriately without undue guilt.
6. They can abandon overprotective or unduly harsh behavioral patterns toward their child.

Drotar, Baskiewicz, Irvin, Kenell, and Klaus (1975) referred to this final stage as "reorganization," in which positive, long-term acceptance has developed and guilt has lessened.

In applying these stages, the professional needs to be mindful that families are not homogeneous. These stages may not be a good fit for some families. For some, these stages are cyclical and recur as new developmental milestones are achieved, or when a crisis occurs (e.g., a child's condition worsens). For others, although a particular reaction may be the most dominant one, other reactions may also be present (Hornby, 1994). For example, when parents' predominant emotion is anger, they may also be experiencing some denial and sadness. Other factors that affect the manifestations of these stages include whether they may be determined in part by one's culture, whether social support is available (Thompson & Gustafson, 1996), whether all family members experience the same stage at the same time, and how long a particular stage lasts. According to Hornby (1994), "Some parents appear to work the process in a few days, whereas others seem to take years to reach a reasonable level of adaptation. Just as for any major loss it is considered that most people will take around two years to come to terms with the disability. However, some parents seem to take longer and a few possibly never fully adjust to the situation" (p. 20).

CHRONIC SORROW

The second major theoretical view of family adjustment to childhood disability is the position developed by Olshansky (1962) but later embraced by others (Wikler, Wasow, & Hatfield, 1981; Damrosh & Perry, 1989). Olshansky coined the term "chronic sorrow" to connote a longer or perhaps even lifelong sadness brought about by changes in the child and external events, such as school entry. In regard to chronic sorrow, Marsh (1993) writes, "Stage theories generally reflect an assumption of movement toward a final state of closure characterized by acceptance and adjustment. Increasingly, that view has been challenged by clinicians and researchers who have emphasized the continuing emotional upheavals of families, as well as the absence of time-limited sequential movement through a series of stages" (pp. 121–122).

Searle (1978), the father of a child with mental retardation, also takes issue with stage theory by asserting that "the shock, the guilt, the bitterness—never disappear but stay on as a part of the parents' emotional life" (p. 27). The intensity of the experience of chronic sorrow is seen as varying over time and can be influenced not only by the degree or changes in the disability, or by life events, as suggested earlier, but also by the parents' personality, ethnic group identification, religion, and social class. Max (1985) suggested that the reactions such as anger, sadness, and denial are not resolved but become an integral part of the parents' emotional life. This reoccurrence of parental reactions tends to emerge at various transition points in the child's development, such as school entry, the onset of puberty, leaving school, or leaving home (Hornby, 1995). It can also occur when parents are informed about an additional disability at some time subsequent to the initial diagnosis. One parent recounts how having apparently come to terms with her child being blind, she was devastated when mental retardation was later diagnosed (Featherstone, 1980). Firestein (1989) talked about the dreams that can be destroyed by childhood illness/disability, asserting that the sense of lost dreams is chronic and grief is experienced in some measure over many years.

Olshansky (1962) believed chronic sorrow to be a natural response to childhood disability, because unlike families of children without disabilities, these families will not see their children ultimately become self-sufficient adults. We now know that some adult children can function independently; others, as a result of family and community supports are semi-independent; still others remain dependent throughout their lives.

Increased knowledge about family coping and the continuous evolution of community resources have helped to combat the previous lack of family and community support. Key legislative initiatives and the empowerment of family members have contributed to the positive climate that currently exists. Also, parents who do experience sadness about their child's disability can still be competent and caring. Too often, professionals have been quick to label parents as unaccepting or poorly adjusted when they are, in fact, reacting normally to their continuing burden.

From their research, Wikler et al. (1981) reported that parental sorrow appears to be periodic rather than continuous, with the level of intensity related to some of the developmental junctures noted earlier and to the coping abilities of the parents. In another study, mothers and fathers of children with Down syndrome reported that the majority of mothers (68%) experienced peaks and valleys, as well as periodic crises (Damrosh & Perry, 1989). A majority of the fathers (83%), however, depicted their adjustment in terms of steady, gradual recovery. This study suggests that gender difference may affect the response to childhood illness or disability.

The concept of chronic sorrow is reflected in the voices of two parents from Marsh's study (1993, p. 123):

"It is constant grieving throughout our lives. Feelings of frustration because [of] fighting the system and seeing very little progress."

"The pain's there, it never leaves. I am to the point now where I'm kind of over the self-blame part of it. Every once in a while it will crop up. I tried hard to give her the best that I had at the time. I tried to make the best decisions I could for her. Given what I had, what I knew then, I think I've done a good job. But I always think maybe I could have done a little better. So it's painful. I hope the day comes that I can close my eyes and get a little bit of peace."

Before leaving the chronic sorrow theory of adjustment to childhood disability, I want to leave the reader with Olshansky's own words, relative to the view he articulated in 1962: "The permanent, day-by-day dependence of the child, the interminable frustrations resulting from the child's relative changelessness, the unesthetic quality of mental defectiveness, the deep symbolism buried in the process of giving birth to a defective child, all these join together to produce the parent's chronic sorrow" (p. 192).

PSYCHOSOCIAL STRESSES ASSOCIATED WITH CHILDHOOD ILLNESS/DISABILITY

The previous section addressed parental response to the period of time subsequent to diagnosis. Some family members may take longer to reach acceptance, and, as noted earlier, others may experience a mild yet chronic sadness. We now explore five stresses commonly experienced by families as a consequence of chronic childhood illness/disability: intellectual, instrumental, emotional, interpersonal, and existential (Brinthaupt, 1991; Chesler & Barbarin, 1987).

Intellectual stress is mainly associated with the process of gathering initial information, when determining an accurate diagnosis occupies the parents' attention. It is not uncommon for parents of children with certain disorders (e.g., cystic fibrosis, rare and multiple disabilities) to engage in the frustrating process of visiting a number of medical specialists. With some disorders, several misdiagnoses occur before a correct one is given. However, once the diagnosis is made, parents usually experience a compelling need for information (Hobbs, Perrin, & Ireys, 1986).

The parents' quest for information regarding etiology, prognosis, and treatment options helps to enhance their sense of control in a very anxiety-provoking situation. Parents may engage in "doctor shopping," which may make them susceptible to "quack" treatments, although some "shopping" may be necessary to reach a professional who can make a definitive diagnosis.

According to Brinthaupt (1991), various intellectual stresses are imposed on parents as they attempt to comprehend their child's disorder. Parents may be required to integrate vast amounts of information about disease physiology; the timing and type of treatments, and the rationale for them; symptoms of decline or improvement; complications; and side effects of treatment. In writing about childhood cancer, Chesler and Barbarin (1987) observe that "the stress of wondering if they are handling treatments and side effects properly is escalated by the stakes involved—the child's comfort and even life may hang in the balance" (p. 42). Brinthaupt (1991) adds that "the overriding task of learning the skills necessary to effectively operate within a medical subculture is an intellectual stress not to be underestimated for its difficulty as well as importance" (p. 301).

Instrumental stress involves tasks that are necessary to incorporate the child's medical care and treatment into the lifestyle of the family. The goal is to achieve as much equilibrium as possible in the family system. Parents become front-line caregivers and, as a result, become proficient as professionals in the management of their child. While simultaneously attending to their disabled child's needs, they must also be vigilant to the needs of other family members, such as other children or their spouse. Brinthaupt (1991) lists the following instrumental challenges:

1. Financial management.
2. Determining the division of labor in the family so that adequate care is provided for the child with a disability.
3. Accomplishing necessary household chores in addition to caretaking.
4. Becoming aware of signs that indicate a negative impact of the illness on family members.
5. Knowing when and how to seek assistance.
6. Fostering a sense of normalcy despite the demands of the illness/disability.

The financial demands on a family are instrumental stresses that are often given short shrift in the professional literature. Direct medical care, in-home, and self-care expenses, as well as expenses for special diets, special schools, time lost from work, home modifications, and the like, constitute significant sources of stress. Also, one parent, usually the mother, often relinquishes a career in order to remain at home to care for the child. A decision to stay at home necessitates a sacrifice and negates a second income that could help with uninsured expenses. It may also mean that a parent must forego pursuing more challenging or lucrative career opportunities, if such a choice would remove the family from the vicinity of a treatment facility. These financial demands can interfere with potentially restorative and interpersonally rewarding family activities, such as vacations (Brinthaupt, 1991).

Emotional stress encompasses both psychogenic factors and reactive responses to the demands of caregiving. Responses might include lack of sleep, loss of energy, and excessive worry and anxiety (Chesler & Barbarin, 1987). A key factor contributing to the emotional response includes the uncertainty regarding disease prognosis and responses to periodic exacerbation of the illness/disability (Perrin & MacLean, 1988; Jessop & Stein, 1985). Furthermore, the uncertainty and ambiguity that accompany illness/disability can compromise parents' sense of perceived control.

Parents of children with rare disorders can feel isolated, which increases emotional stress, because it is unlikely that they will encounter another family with a child that has the same condition (Seligman & Darling, 1997). Another contributor to emotional stress is the heart-wrenching experience of watching a child suffer and not being able to relieve that suffering. The specter of experiencing a child's death is immobilizing and can leave in its wake a lifelong sadness (Sourkes, 1982). Also, heightened vigilance for signs of relapse or disease exacerbation can add to stress and anxiety.

Interpersonal stress can follow on the heels of pediatric disability/illness. Interpersonal stress can involve family members, friends, and medical or educational personnel. Although divorce rates among these families are virtually equivalent to families in which there is no illness/disability (Kalins, 1983; Sabbeth & Leventhal, 1984; Brinthaupt, 1991; Seligman & Darling, 1997), there does appear to be evidence of marital distress for some families (Moorman, 1992; Siegel & Silverstein, 1994; McHugh, 1999). More research is needed to clarify the role of marital distress in these families compared to families with non-disabled children. Brinthaupt (1991) speculates that marital distress may not necessarily be maladaptive. Perhaps, at times, it may serve an adaptive function; for some, it may lead to seeking help from a mental health professional (Laborde & Seligman, 1991). There is some suggestion, however, that high-recurrent-risk diseases serve as a threat to marital stability.

Brinthaupt (1991) observed that the incidence of divorce in families in which a child has a nonhereditary disorder (e.g., leukemia) or a low-recurrence disability (e.g., spine bifida) is lower than the national average, whereas the divorce rate in families with a high-recurrence-risk illness (e.g., cystic fibrosis) is comparable to the national average. It is important to acknowledge once again that marital distress in some families may be more related to problems the marital partners have with each other than with the child who has the disability. I wrote about this issue in a chapter in Don Meyer's (1995) book, *Uncommon Fathers: Reflections on Raising a Child with a Disability:*

> I believe that one needs to be careful about the relationship between marital conflict or divorce to the presence of a child with special needs. The decision to dissolve a marriage is a complex one, made up of personal styles and values, family of origin issues, external factors, and the like. My suspicion is that the general public believes that a child with a disability creates enormous tensions within the family, eventually culminating in divorce. On the other hand, parents who speak and write about their experiences with their child project the notion that a child with a disability marshals constructive forces within the family system and eventually brings family members together. My guess is that the truth probably falls somewhere between what the general public seems to believe and what some parents have projected in their public utterances and in their writings. We need to openly address this issue so that the public is better informed and that parents who have experienced divorce are not filled with guilt and shame due to the perception that most families are actually brought closer. (Seligman, 1995, pp. 178–179)

Interpersonal distress can appear in other family members as well because non-disabled children and extended family members are also affected by childhood disability, a topic that will be explored more fully later in this chapter. Finally, interpersonal stress can emerge from potentially stressful encounters with the public (Wikler, 1981; Siegel, 1996). Depending upon the extent to which parents "go public" with their child's disability, they must negotiate the sometimes stressful and awkward transactions with strangers.

Existential stress refers to the family's ability to construct an explanatory meaning framework for its experience. Childhood disability is an affront to an assumed developmental order of the family life cycle. "Childhood is supposed to be a time of well-being, or, at worst, a period of self-limited, transitory illness, and not a time of threats to viability or function" (Stein & Jessop, 1984, p. 194). Parents grapple with such existential issues as "Why me?" or "Why my family?" (Kushner, 1981; Seligman, 1979). Cherished notions about God, fate, and a just world are challenged (Chesler & Barbarin, 1987). "If the child is seen as a divine gift, the unexpressed question, 'why did this happen to me?' has the corollary 'why did He do this to me?' and raises the age-old philosophical question, 'If God is good He would not have done this' " (Ross, 1964, p. 62).

A child with a disability may be perceived as a reflection of the mother's adequacy. In situations where a child is viewed as salvaging an unstable marriage, the birth of a child with a disability may be another indication that the marriage is doomed to failure. On the other hand, the infant may be seen as a divine gift, a sign of grace (Ross, 1964). Such a child may be viewed as a sign of special grace because only the most worthy parents would be entrusted with his or her care. One study showed that an ability to endow the child's illness with meaning and a sense of optimism seems to characterize high-functioning families (Venter, 1981).

Some parents appear to be able to explain their child's disorder within the framework of a particular life philosophy, while others alter or abandon their prior religious–spiritual commitments. It is apparent that existential stresses are a formidable challenge for parents of children with chronic illnesses or disabilities (Brinthaupt, 1991).

MARITAL ADJUSTMENT, DIVORCE, AND SINGLE PARENTHOOD

A growing population of single parents in society in general and single parents of children with disabilities appear to experience greater stresses than parents in two-parent families (Vadasy, 1986; Simpson, 1996). In regard to parents of children with autism, Siegel (1996) is unequivocal in her position that single parenthood presents enormous challenges. A particular danger is the possibility that healthy children may become parentified siblings. "In the absence of an adult helpmate, mothers, often without realizing it, depend a great deal on help from the autistic child's brothers and sisters. Seeing a three-year-old take her autistic five-year-old brother firmly by the hand as they are about to cross a busy street gives a picture of how much the life of the three-year-old can be affected by having an autistic sibling" (Siegel, 1996, pp. 139–140). Yet, as noted earlier, most of the assumptions about single parenthood and childhood disability are intuitive; empirical data are scarce. Also, when considering divorce and single parenthood, one needs to bear in mind that divorce does not have the same impact on all family members, that the effects of divorce may depend on when it occurs in the family life cycle and the degree of dysfunction in the family before marital breakup (Schulz, 1987; Simpson, 1996). Furthermore, one cannot necessarily assume that the parents are not involved with their child after a divorce. It is possible that divorced parents can devote more time to their child once the issues that led to the dissolution of their marriage are resolved.

One outcome of divorce exists in families in which one or both parents in the original family remarry (Visher & Visher, 1988). New rules and roles need to be adopted, loyalty issues to the biological and nonbiological parents need to be negotiated, new lines of authority needs to be established, financial responsibilities may need to be reconsidered, and the like. When a child with a disability resides in a blended family, caretaking and primary responsibility for the child need to be negotiated, among other issues.

As suggested earlier, information regarding marital problems and divorce in families of children with disabilities is sparse and contradictory (Crnic et al., 1983; Patterson, 1991; McHugh, 1999). Gabel, McDowell, and Cerreto (1983) report that the onset of marital difficulties is one of the more frequently reported adjustment problems. Their research review shows that marital problems include more frequent conflict, feelings of marital dissatisfaction, sexual difficulties, temporary separations, and divorce. Siegel (1996) estimates that for families of children with disabilities, the divorce rate is about 20% higher than in families with nondisabled children. In his landmark study conducted 40 years ago, Farber (1959) found marital conflict to be common, especially in families containing a retarded boy aged 9 or older. Conversely, some families of children with disabilities report problems no more frequently than comparison families (Bernard, 1974; Dorner, 1975; Martin, 1975; Waisbren, 1980; Patterson, 1991), and some marriages have reportedly improved after the diagnosis of a child's disability (Schwab, 1989). Conclusions about divorce rates among parents with or without a child with disabilities are affected by the presumptions researchers make about divorce rates. Some report that one-half of such marriages end in divorce, while others cite figures closer to one-third.

Although the data regarding marital satisfaction and divorce in families of children with disabilities are contradictory, we do know that some stressed marriages remain intact, others simply fail, while still others survive and thrive. The task of researchers should be to understand why some families do well while others do poorly. Some researchers believe that future investigations should differentiate the child and family characteristics and other ecological factors that distinguish families that cope well and survive from those that do not (Crnic et al., 1983).

As noted earlier, a family's focus on the child with a disability as a source of family problems may in fact be a "red herring" that leads the parents away from more fundamental issues about their relationship (Harris, 1983). It is important that professionals discriminate between family problems related to the stress of coping with childhood disability and those that would have arisen under any circumstances. However, problematic marital relationships can be made considerably worse by the birth of a child with a disability. It is a myth that such a child, or any child for that matter, can improve a troubled marriage (Lederer & Jackson, 1968).

Siegel (1996) noted that parental adjustment to childhood disability may be related to whether a child was planned for and/or desired. She also observed that parents who have planned having children very carefully often experience a greater sense of "unfairness" at having a child with a disability when they compare themselves to others who live their lives in a less planful way. Furthermore, younger couples appear to be able to cope somewhat better than older couples. Their lifestyle preferences are not as fixed, they can decide to have more children, and more physical energy is available to them.

After a thorough review of the literature on families of children with severe disabilities, Lyon and Lyon (1991) concluded that although these families must contend with a number of stressors, in general, the research reveals mixed conclusions regarding the impact of a child with severe disabilities on the family. As other contributors to the literature have observed, these authors also note the major methodological problems inherent in much of the existing research and conclude that in the absence of clear evidence that these families are coping badly, professionals should focus on such practical matters as concrete information, respite services, financial help, and other supportive services to help with practical and logistical problems. In addition, other researchers make a case for providing psychotherapeutic services for some families (Marsh, 1993; Elman, 1991; Laborde & Seligman, 1991; Siegel, 1996).

From this overview, what can we conclude about marital harmony–dysfunction among families of children with disabilities? One conclusion may be that marital dysfunction may have occurred even without the presence of disability. Still another is that in some families, a child with disabilities may aggravate latent problems. Perhaps an acceptable conclusion is that many families can cope successfully with the help of family and community supports.

FAMILIES OF CHILDREN
WITH DIFFERENT DISABILITIES

Although research, observations, and personal accounts of family members of children with different disabling conditions are increasing, the available research is, again, too contradictory to draw any definitive conclusions. Nevertheless, there are some reports of children with dissimilar disabilities that provide a glimpse of the concerns families face. For example, the unpredictable behavior of some autistic children and the social–interpersonal ramifications experienced by their families can cause considerable stress (Bristol, 1984; Schopler & Messibov, 1984; Harris, 1994; Siegel, 1996). Even as we learn more about the biological-bases of certain conditions, parents of children with autism and schizophrenia (albeit very different conditions) are still often considered responsible for the child's illness and thereby suffer the social stigma that accompanies this disorder. Schizophrenia was initially based on a flawed theory of family interaction that was not based on scientific evidence (Dawes, 1994). For families with children who have autism, the high-risk factors include ambiguity of diagnosis, severity and duration of the illness, and lack of congruity with community norms (Bristol, 1984). Cantwell and Baker (1984) cite research indicating that families are affected by the multiple failures of their autistic children. Mothers appear the most affected, and spousal affectional bonds tend to be weakened; siblings also are affected, and family difficulties do not diminish as the child grows older.

The unpredictability of seizures among children with epilepsy may result in family members' constant vigilance for seizure activity (Lechtenberg, 1984). Public attitudes toward persons with epilepsy resemble the attitudes toward persons with mental illness, thereby creating a major stressor for the family. Families with a hemophilic child need to be constantly vigilant of their child's bleeding episodes, and families of children with heart disease need to be cautious about bringing home infections (Travis, 1976). All of these characteristics of the child's disability may cause stress in the family and precipitate major family crisis when other family problems exist. As Tartar (1987) points out, the contribution of the parents' characteristics, together with the demand characteristics of the child's disability, "underscores again the complex dynamic and reciprocal relationship between parent and offspring with the characteristics of one affecting the reactions of the other" (p. 83).

As with most disabling conditions, the effect of a deaf child on the family is mixed (Luterman, 1984). However, hearing-impaired children often also have impaired communication, which can be a source of considerable frustration for family members (Sloman, Springer, & Vachon, 1993). Fewell (1991) reports that the degree of visual loss in blind children has important implications for the child and the family's reaction to him or her. Just as children with low vision try to "pass" as normally sighted, parents, too, are caught in the dilemma of not wanting to identify their children's differences. Although children who are blind may struggle with mobility, and there is some evidence of delayed and aberrant social behavior, the fact that a blind child can think, communicate, and carry on with the chores of daily living may make blindness less devastating to the blind child and the family than other disabilities (Fewell, 1991).

For children with physical disabilities, mobility is most affected, which, depending upon the severity of the disability may affect their ability to perform self-care functions. However, as with most conditions, psychological and social factors are directly tied to the disability. For example, persons with a physical disability may shrink from interactions with nondisabled peers, fearing their negative response (Marshak & Seligman, 1993). By isolating oneself from others, a person may become despondent. Physical impairments can take a variety of forms, such as loss of limbs or a paralysis due to accident or disease. The nature, characteristics, and severity of the physical impairment may determine the type of adjustment the child and the family must make (Marshak & Seligman, 1993). For example, caring for a child with quadripelegia has numerous implications for how family members contribute to frequent caretaking duties. In the case of a child with muscular dystrophy, a degenerative disease, the child and family need to adjust to an increasing level of dependency as the disease progresses. Numerous other physical disorders, many of which are rare and leave the family with few others with whom to identify, may cause problems for the family.

Mullins (1979) reports that the physical needs of children with cancer affect the entire family: "The medications, hospitalizations, repeated transportation for treatment, and extended care at home will be a drain on family finances and physical resources" (p. 266). If the cancer is terminal, the family needs to prepare for the child's imminent death (Sourkes, 1982). This can be a crisis of major proportions and requires considerable family adjustment before and after the child's death occurs.

Cystic fibrosis, one of the most common chronic diseases of childhood, requires the family to comply with a prescribed home regimen. This disease, resulting in pulmonary dysfunction, also involves the pancreatic and gastrointestinal systems, and presents serious challenges for the coping skills and adjustment of the family (Brinthaupt, 1991). The home care of the child is difficult and chronic, and failure to carry out treatment can contribute to the progression of the disease and eventual death (Dushenko, 1981). Communication in these families often declines in a situation that is difficult and requires the continued expression of hope and mutual support (Patterson, 1985). McCracken (1984) reports that families of children with cystic fibrosis have multiple problems, and Offer, Ostrov, and Howard (1984) argue that problems of an adolescent with cystic fibrosis are exacerbated by short stature and the appearance of lower maturational level. Social stigma, as noted earlier, adds to the disability.

It is impossible to conclude with any certainty how the type of disability will affect the family. Factors other than type may play an important role in determining family adaptation (Crnic et al., 1983). We know from Rolland (1993) that onset, course, prognosis, as well as other illness/disability-related variables may influence family response. Researchers report that the quantity and quality of community resources and family support have an impact on the family's ability to cope with childhood disability (Wortis & Margolies, 1955; Korn, Chess, & Fernandez, 1978; Darling, 1991). Researchers have sought to determine how and which aspects of social support are most helpful to families (Kazak & Marvin, 1984; Kazak & Wilcox, 1984; Krahn, 1993).

According to one study, mothers of children with disabilities experience significantly more stress if their offspring have a greater number of, or unusual, caregiving demands, are less socially responsive, have more difficult temperaments, and display more repetitive behavioral patterns (Beckman, 1983). Beckman's research is important in that it represents a departure from other studies by examining specific child characteristics rather than medical labels. Beckman's results support those of Tartar (1987) and the observations of Siegel and Silverstein (1994), who report that it is the behavioral aspects of a condition that are most distressing to the family.

In a study of 111 parents of children with hemophilia, researchers found that the parental burden caused by their child's illness was rather small (Varekamp et al., 1990). In fact, 45% of the parents reported that their marriages had improved compared with 4% who felt that their marriages had worsened. With hemophilia, bleeding is mostly unexpected and requires immediate attention. The risk of bleeding creates for parents an internal struggle between wanting to protect the child and also wanting to avoid limiting the child's independence. This appears to be less problematic to parents than dealing with children who isolate themselves, do not communicate, have outbursts, and experience behavior problems (Harris, 1994).

In the face of inclusive research data, it is important to be cognizant of the numerous variables that may affect family adjustment and to persuade professionals to keep these variables in mind when evaluating a family's level of functioning.

MOTHERS, FATHERS, SIBLINGS, AND THE EXTENDED FAMILY

Much of what we know about childhood disability and the family comes from research on mothers. More recently, however, studies have included fathers. There is also a growing number of studies on siblings and a modest literature on grandparents. The following section briefly reviews these family roles, starting with mothers.

Mothers

It is inevitable that a mother about to give birth has a host of expectations, not the least of which is the anticipation of a child with all the attributes of normality that will enable the child to assume the roles generally ascribed by society. Although expectations vary, depending on a multiplicity of factors, mothers expect their children to achieve at least as much as they have been able to accomplish in their lifetime. Writing of parental reactions to children born with severe brain defects, Baum (1962) cites Kozier in observing:

> In many ways, a child represents to the parent an extension of his own self. . . . When the baby is born, the mother's wish to be loved is partially transferred from her own person to that of the baby. To the father, a normal child is often an affirmation, at least in part, of his sense of success. The capacity to produce unimpaired offspring is psycho-

logically and culturally important for the parents' sense of personal adequacy. (p. 335)

More recently, Judy O'Halloran (1993) writes about an exchange between herself and her pediatrician shortly after the birth of her son Casey, who has Down syndrome:

> I remember his asking, "How do you plan to raise Casey? Do you plan to do anything differently than you did with Sean and Ryan?" That seemed to be a strange question, but since we'd known each other a long time and since he seemed to be in this psychological mode, I didn't give it much thought.
>
> "Gosh, Irwin [the pediatrician] he's the third one. I'm an old hand at this. I'm sure I'll be a lot easier on him. Besides, Sean and Ryan are 180° apart in personality. Casey has to fit somewhere in between. So raising him will be a piece of cake."
>
> A few minutes later, Irwin put Casey back in my arms. Then with tears in his eyes, he said, "I strongly suspect Casey has Down syndrome."
>
> CRASH! Our world fell apart. And with it crumbles all that confidence. (p. 20)

In terms of one's personal sense of adequacy, Featherstone (1980), from her inspired book, *A Difference in the Family*. writes that: "Participants in a mothers' group—discuss, without a startling sense of novelty or revelation, the fear that their children's handicaps are somehow their faults. Their self-esteem has plummeted, and they know why" (p. 72).

The ritual of counting fingers and toes shortly after birth reflects many mothers' underlying fear that their infants may have been born with disabilities. Although this fear is expressed in subtle and camouflaged ways, the belief that "It can't happen to me" is also present. When parents' expectations of a healthy, "normal" child are contradicted by the birth of an infant with disabilities, their coping abilities are put to the test. Coping tends to be a complicated process and the effects on parents of coping with childhood disability may be both cyclical and cumulative.

According to one review of the literature (Thompson & Gustafson, 1996), mothers of children with various disabilities, who were compared to control mothers with healthy children, fared essentially the same on measures of depression, stress, social isolation, alcohol problems, and similar research indices. There was some suggestion that mothers of children with a psychiatric disability fared less well, and that mothers generally did well when they perceived support from their husbands and other sources.

The more immediate biological role of the mother in the birth process may endow the discrepancy between expectation and reality with greater psychological meaning for her than for her husband, at least initially. At the time of first information, it is the mother who may experience severe feelings of guilt, remorse, and lowered self-esteem.

Although it is not entirely clear whether or how the birth of an infant with a disability affects mothers and fathers differently, the shock renders both parents physically and psychologically vulnerable. During this period, a mother's (as well as father's) ability to recognize, evaluate, and adapt to the newly encountered situation is often compromised. Of course, some disabilities are not detectable at birth but may become manifest as a child fails to complete developmental tasks. In retrospect, after discovering their child's exceptionality months or even years after birth, mothers may admit that they suspected rather early that their child was "different." For example, after a diagnosis has been communicated, a mother of a newborn with retardation may say that she secretly suspected something was wrong because her son was not as active in the womb as her other child. Another potential reaction from mothers is to experience a premonition, such as the one described by Trainer (1991), while picnicking in the park with her family:

> Somebody was entering the park, up the wooded pathway to the picnic grove. Four children and two women were walking very slowly, too slowly. As they came near I saw that the children were severely retarded. I winced inwardly. Why oh why did they have to come to the park on this particular day?
>
> I watched as they made their way slowly along the path and disappeared among the redwoods. I had never before that day laid eyes upon those children. And yet, deep within me it was as if memory rang a distant bell, as if somehow I knew them. Or would come to know them.
>
> Why oh why had they come to the park on this particular day?
>
> Two years later our fourth child was born and we were told that he had Down syndrome. Only they didn't call it Down syndrome then; they called it Mongolism. Ben, our cherubic baby, was a Mongoloid and we were no longer observers in the park. (pp. 1, 3)

In regard to mothers' guilt over giving birth to a child with a disability, Featherstone (1980) believes that mothers take great pride or assume the burden of their offsprings accomplishments and characteristics: "The whole culture supports a mother in the opinion that her children are what she has made them. Whether from upbringing, Freud, or *Family Circle*, most women learn the lesson thoroughly by the time they are grown" (p. 71).

Featherstone refers to a saying from old Boston pols that if you take credit for the sunshine, then you are going to have to shoulder the blame for snow. Moreover, she believes that because fathers spend more time away from the home than mothers, they spend fewer hours with their children and thus play a secondary role in child development and, hence, take less credit for it. Featherstone asserts that mothers are particularly vulnerable when a child has a disability. She believes that even if a mother works, her happiness and her sense of achievement are more closely tied than her husband's to her children's physical and emotional well-being.

Even though mothers, in Featherstone's opinion, are more vulnerable at birth or at diagnosis, they are simultaneously more fortunate in that they are more likely than their husbands to realize just how shattered they are.

> My own impression (based on the accounts of parents and on countless conversations with them) is that while the father of a handicapped child usually recognizes the practical problems of care, his wife's suffering, his own sadness, embarrassment, rage, and even despair, he is less attuned to the possibility that his own self-confidence has suffered. And maybe it has not: in the eyes of the world, a man's major accomplishments are outside the family. Nevertheless, some fathers do report feelings of guilt. I would guess that self-doubt nags others as well. (Featherstone, 1980, p. 72)

Fathers

With the historical emphasis on mothers and attachment, the role of fathers in child development and family functioning has been undervalued. Although there have been marked changes in gender roles, men and women historically have been cast into somewhat rigid instrumental and expressive roles. The relaxation of sex role in society has enabled some family members to respond more flexibly to changing family needs. As a result of increased role flexibility, fathers are more willing to adopt nurturing roles and also now considered capable alternative caregivers for children. Furthermore, they have more time to spend with their children due to the shortening of the work week, home-based businesses, and flex-time schedules (Pruett, 1987). Although there are differences in the way fathers and mothers interact with their children, both parents are now accepted as competent nurturers and caretakers (Lamb & Meyer, 1991).

There is only a modest research base on fathers of children with disabilities and some of the studies that exist have been compromised in a number of ways (Marsh, 1992; Lamb & Meyer, 1991; Hornby, 1995). However, some information is available from the research and personal accounts of fathers' experiences.

It seems that fathers and mothers initially respond differently to the news that they are parents of a child with a disability. Fathers tend to respond less emotionally at the time of diagnosis and focus on long-term concerns, whereas mothers respond more emotionally and are concerned about their ability to cope with the burdens of child care. Generally speaking, fathers seem more concerned than mothers about the adoption of socially acceptable behavior by their children—especially their sons—and they are more anxious about the social status and occupational success of their offspring (Lamb & Meyer, 1991).

Because of the high expectations fathers have of their sons, they may be particularly disappointed when they have a boy with a disability (Farber, 1959; Grossman, 1972). As a result, some fathers manifest with their sons extremes of intense involvement and total withdrawal, and they seem to have limited, routine involvement with their daughters who are disabled (Chigier, 1972; Tallman, 1965; Grossman, 1972). A later study does not support this conclusion, suggesting that more research is needed in this area (Houser & Seligman, 1991). McHugh (1999) writes about why fathers are moved to withdraw from the family: "What makes so many fathers withdraw from the grisly dailiness of caring for their child with multiple physical and mental problems? So often they just aren't there. They try, but it is often easier to escape into work or drinking, or bowling, or something to get them out of the house" (p. 56).

Fathers' reactions to their children with disabilities may have implications for the other family members. One study found a high relationship between the degree of paternal acceptance of the child and the amount of acceptance and rejection generally observed in the home (Peck & Stephens, 1960). Not only is the development of the child with a disability likely to be affected when fathers choose to withdraw, but the entire family suffers. As the father withdraws, the burden of care generally falls on other family members, particularly the mother.

A problem for some fathers is their discomfort with strong emotions. Men are supposed to "fix" things, to be stoic and in charge (Smith, 1981). Having a child with a disability is a profound challenge for some fathers who ascribe to traditional male values and as a result may suffer more than their spouses from having a child with a disability (Seligman & Darling, 1997).

A father's stoic behavior can be viewed by professionals as a more manageable reaction. The male physicians quoted below seem to feel more comfortable communicating distressing information to fathers than to mothers:

> Usually I prefer to tell the father. The mother is in an emotional state after having just given birth.
>
> Usually, I tell the father, and, based on his knowledge of his wife, we decide on a course of action. . . . I do this for psychological reasons. My feeling is that you can deal more easily with the father. It's emotionally easier.
>
> If I had a choice, I'd probably prefer talking with the father first and let him help me make the decision about talking to the mother.
>
> I call the father and ask him what he wants me to do. I wait until I can reach the father before I talk to the mother.
>
> I try to talk to the obstetrician to find out if it's the mother's first baby or if she's anxious or apprehensive. . . . I always tell the father right away. (Darling, 1979, p. 206)

In his fathers' discussion groups, Smith (1981) found that group members distrusted male displays of emotion and that the fathers learned as children that "real men" are always in control of their emotions, that "Big boys don't cry." Smith believes that these masculine behaviors place considerable stress on the father and make it harder for him to express and be attuned to his own feelings.

> For men in the fathers' discussion groups, these facets of the stereotypic masculine role were quite restrictive and presented obstacles to the men's coming to terms with their children's handicaps and with their own feelings as parents to exceptional children. In particular, these men displayed stereotypical instrumental traits such as a reluctance to show one's emotions, a need for independence and self-reliance, and a need to "fix" problematic situations. (p. 12)

Smith points out that, as fathers of children with disabilities, these men experienced a variety of intense emotions that they could not easily express or confront. For example, many felt anger at the physicians who initially informed them of their child's disability, believing that these doctors were unnecessarily abrupt and unsympathetic. Furthermore, the fathers found themselves dependent on the expertise of professionals. This dependence was difficult for the fathers because it made them feel less in control and less competent as parents. As noted, males grow up to be "fixers" who actively confront problems. Passivity in the face of a crisis is threatening to men who have learned that they must be "strong," avoid showing weakness (mainly by suppressing emotions), and be able to resolve difficult situations competently. Perhaps the most poignant frustration is that fathers simply cannot "fix" their child's disability.

For most of the fathers, involvement in the discussion groups represented the first time they had acknowledged to anyone—to their wives or even to themselves—that the birth of their child had resulted in such strong feelings.

Adjusting to a child with a disability can be a considerable challenge to fathers. Some become engulfed in depression, while others grow from the experience. Talking about his deaf, blind, and paralyzed daughter, one father offered the following personal insight: "Jessica has taught me what true love is. Poets and preachers, young lovers, and idealists have professed knowledge of this elusive concept for years. But in Jessica's silence, I have learned the real essence of love: you give everything and expect nothing in return" (Dale, 1995, p. 2).

Another father of a son with multiple disabilities offered his perspective:

> If I were to offer advice to other fathers of children with disabilities, I would encourage them to be pragmatic. Realize that others will only understand part of your being and few will understand the road you must travel. Keep something for yourself—don't define your life in terms of your child. To do so will eat away at your health, both physical and mental. (Dixon, 1995, p. 122)

Josh Greenfeld (1978) describes the powerful and contradictory feelings he experiences as he reflects on life with his autistic son, Noah:

> I thought continually that soon I will have to kill Noah. The monster that has long been lurking in him increasingly shows its face. And just as the day may come when I can no longer bear to take care of him, I could not bear to see him mistreated—or maltreated—in a state hospital like Camarillo or Lechworth Village.

He will become a hopeless grotesque with less than endearing manners. He keeps putting his fingers to his lips and then spit-touching the nearest object or person. He pinches, he scratches, he pulls hair. This morning he suddenly pulled Foumi's [Greenfeld's wife] hair after she had chastised him for his finger-spitting. I heard her crying and rushed to free her from his grasp.

Killing him would be a kindness. His brain has stopped working; he has not been functioning anyway. I dread it but I see myself killing my son not as a myth but as a fact. My dreams now are dreams of prison. Isolation. A winding down of my life in solitude. It seems absurd, I know. But could I ever bear to see Noah suffer, killed softly day after day? No.

Noah is quick to scream, to clutch, to demand, to be unreasonable. He is a tyranny I will never quite learn to live with. He is an obsession I will never learn to live without. (pp. 94–95)

In spite of these negative indicators of fathers' ability to adapt to childhood disability, there are fathers who cope well and in fact become involved in helping other fathers come to grips with their special circumstances (Meyer, 1995). One example of this is the fathers' program that began in 1978 at the University of Washington (Meyer, Vadasy, Fewell, & Schell, 1985). This program has become national in scope as fathers and professional facilitators are being trained to provide workshops for fathers of children with disabilities. The workshops integrate discussions with information and opportunities for fathers to learn how to socialize and play with their sons and daughters who are disabled.

The research from these workshops is encouraging. One study reported that fathers experience lower stress and depression and higher satisfaction levels than parents newly entering the program (Vadasy, Fewell, Meyer, & Greenberg, 1985). Another evaluation of 45 sets of parents found that both mothers and fathers reported significantly decreased depression, and fathers had a decrease in stress and grief (Vadasy, Fewell, Greenberg, Desmond, & Meyer, 1986).

Fathers have a need for information about their children's disability, programs, services, and treatment options that is equal to that of mothers (Darling & Baxter, 1996; Seligman, 1995). It is important that organizations and educational institutions serving children with disabilities encourage the involvement of fathers and include them in their programs.

In his book, *Uncommon Fathers: Reflections on Raising a Child with a Disability*, Meyer (1995), edited a series of poignant essays by fathers on their experiences of parenting a child, adolescent, or young adult with a disability. The contributing fathers reflect considerable diversity in background: a rabbi, a retired police officer, a few attorneys, a Christian missionary, a parole officer, authors, and college professors. In the preface, Meyer writes that "the opinions and experiences of fathers of children with special needs are anything but monolithic. As might be expected from such a diverse group of men, the authors hold differing religious and philosophical interpretations of their children's disabilities. They possess a wide range of coping strategies. Some are upbeat and optimistic; others are still struggling; most are somewhere in between" (p. vii). Although research is essential to understanding a father's reaction to his child's disability, there is a richness and depth of understanding that appears in personal essays that cannot be replicated by research data.

Siblings

Until recently, siblings constituted the forgotten family member (Siegel & Silverstein, 1994). However, in the late 1960s and the 1970s, there was a trickle of research devoted to sibling adjustment to having an ill or disabled brother or sister. The 1980s and 1990s witnessed a surge of interest in sibling adjustment, as evidenced by the spate of books devoted to the subject (Powell & Gallagher, 1993; Stoneman & Berman, 1993; Siegel & Silverstein, 1994; Meyer & Vadasy, 1994; Harris, 1994; Moorman, 1992; Fanos, 1996; Neugeboren, 1997; McHugh, 1999). Sibling relationships are often the longest and most enduring of family relationships. As Powell and Gallagher (1993) noted: "Siblings provide a continuing relationship from which there is no annulment" (p. 14).

Speaking about children with chronic or fatal illnesses, Fanos (1996) reports:

> The emerging incidence of chronic illness in youngsters poses serious psychosocial challenges. Many different chronic and/or fatal illnesses afflict young people, with resultant effects on their families, including their well brothers and sisters. Technological advances, pharmaceutical treatments, and earlier diagnoses have allowed children with serious illnesses to live into their teens and beyond. An appreciation of the enormity of the impact on the family and the well siblings has not kept pace with such remarkable medical breakthroughs. Although the severity of the impact on siblings is beginning to be acknowledged in the literature, there has been little understanding of exactly how exposure

to chronic illness and death of a sibling generates subsequent difficulties. (p. xi)

Being the brother or sister of a child with a chronic illness or disability constitutes a risk factor for some nondisabled siblings. Siblings who are expected to provide care for a brother–sister with a disability may show signs of resentment, anger, and rebelliousness—and guilt at having such feelings.

> I first encountered illness in my family when I was nine years old. My sister Beatriz, who was seven at the time, developed a severe case of Bell's palsy, a neurological condition that is much more serious in children than in adults. Her face became markedly disfigured, and she had a lot of difficulties eating and drinking. Since she could not close one of her eyes and developed a corneal abrasion, her eye needed to be taped down several times during the day and night. Doctors recommended that Beatriz be protected from all potential stressors, including any form of discipline.
>
> Almost immediately after her illness invaded our lives, many demands for cooperation and new caretaking responsibilities were hoisted upon me. In addition to protecting Beatriz, I was targeted to bear the brunt of all discipline and criticism. My mother's increasing irritation and bad moods were also more likely to be deflected onto me. As a result, I rebelled against her and ignited arguments that fueled the spirals of conflict to new heights. My father tried to mediate and insisted that my first duty was to help and cooperate with my mother, who "had enough problems." (Falicov, 1997, pp. 48–49)

One sometimes finds an ambivalent relationship between disabled and nondisabled children due to powerful and conflicted feelings of love, obligation, anger, and resentment. Some siblings feel that their lives are "on hold" while they and their family pool their resources to take care of the ill or disabled family member.

"One particularly guilt-making cause of anger is noticing that a lot of the money available in the family is going to take care of the brother or sister with a disability. If anything can make you feel selfish and greedy, it's resentment of the family's resources pouring into the medical, educational, and therapeutic needs of the child with the disability. You feel like a thoroughly bad person, and when you're a child, you don't know that you aren't bad" (McHugh, 1999, p. 67).

A key variable in how troubled the nondisabled sibling is depends on how the parents handle the situation. A particularly toxic situation occurs when parents expect a child to continuously care for a brother–sister with a disability, while at the same time neglecting his or her needs. Modest and appropriate caretaking accompanied by parental attention (love, concern, support, and guidance) provide a sound foundation for the nondisabled children. In the absence of appropriate parenting, Siegel (1996) estimates that about 50% of siblings view their childhood as compromised in some substantial way by the stresses associated with the presence of their sibling. The remaining 50% feel more neutral about the experience or believe that it has actually helped them. The yearning for parental attention is reflected in the following words by Mary McHugh:

> I yearned for her love as a child. She praised every sound, every physical move, every tiny step forward my brother made. I wanted her to praise me, too. I wanted her to lavish extravagant praise on me for my A report cards, for the stories I wrote that were published in the school newspaper, for the puppet shows I wrote and directed, for my talent as a writer. I tried harder and harder to please her. The one time she did say something fairly positive to me, I treasured her words and remember them to this day. (1999, p. 117)

Age-appropriate information helps young children understand their brother or sister's condition (Seligman & Darling, 1997; Powell & Gallagher, 1993; McHugh, 1999). Ambiguity about a child's disability creates fear and anxiety about the transmissibility of a condition, how long it will last, whether it is a taboo topic within the confines of the family, and whether the well sibling may actually have caused the disability.

Some believe that excessive caretaking, parental inattention, and lack of open communication in the family provide the foundation for serious psychological problems in the adult siblings' life (Siegel & Silverstein, 1994). And since these relationships are lifelong, siblings' involvement with their brother or sister may actually become intensified during adulthood (Moorman, 1992; Neugeboren, 1997; McHugh, 1999). Adult siblings worry about caretaking duties as they and their disabled siblings enter middle and old age. Some single siblings wonder if a prospective spouse will be accepting of a brother–sister with a disability. Furthermore, nondisabled siblings may worry about the social stigma from which their parents may have shielded them.

An interesting by-product of having a brother or sister with a disability in the context of a caring and understanding family is the values one develops that can effect career decisions. Some siblings, especially those who have had positive family experiences, internalize helping values that move them to contribute to the welfare of others and toward life goals that require dedication and sacrifice, such as medicine, special education, and social work (Seligman & Darling, 1997; Siegel, 1996). However, there is some recent research that questions this assertion. For example, Konstam et al. (1993) found that college-age students with and without brothers–sisters with disabilities projected career goals that were divided somewhat equally between service and non-service-oriented careers.

Siegel (1996) believes that siblings exhibit discernible patterns of coping that are reflected in certain roles that these children adopt. As an illustration, the *parentified child* is a fairly common role that siblings assume as caretaking issues inevitably emerge in the family. These children act more like parents than brothers and sisters to their siblings with a disability. They become the "keepers" instead of the "kept." Some parentified children may accept this role with little adverse affect, while others may be resentful and feel guilty about their resentfulness. Also, parents and professionals working with families should be aware that parentification can deprive children of their own childhood. It is important that siblings have opportunities to be children. McHugh (1999) offers an interesting personal perspective on the caretaking role some siblings adopt:

> My own marriage has changed over the years. I was very much a people-pleasing caretaker at first, partly because most women were like that in the fifties. When I learned to stand up for myself, our marriage improved and I changed into what Julia Tallard Johnson calls a "caregiver"—the healthy version of the caretaker. Caregivers take care of themselves first even while they provide support and nurturing to others. . . . They are able to end relationships that are a threat to their psychological, spiritual, or physical well-being. (p. 228)

Some siblings do not try to earn parental attention by helping. Instead, they may become *withdrawn children*. They may be overwhelmed by parental demands for help or driven away by their disabled brother–sister's behavior. Siegel notes that, often, withdrawn children are younger siblings who have never had much attention from their parents. These children are slow to warm up to new situations and usually are not very gregarious. "With the added stress of minimally available parenting, they psychologically give up" (1996,

p. 152). Withdrawn children can benefit from individual and group counseling.

The *superachiever, or family mascot*, compensates for the loss that family members experience. When one child is disabled, parents feel better about their circumstances if another child is developing normally, or, even better, is an exceptional achiever. Sometimes, too much is expected of the other child when the parents' goals for that child exceed his or her abilities. Just like the parentified child, the superachieving child realizes that by succeeding in activities that the parents value, he or she can garner their attention. Siegel (1996) notes that many parentified children are also high achievers. The "mascot," who may not be academically or otherwise talented, tries hard to establish an identity to which parents pay attention, such as using humor or being a show-off.

The *withdrawn child* becomes isolated from family life. Very withdrawn children should be seen by a psychologist to evaluate why they have adopted this strategy. Siegel (1996) finds both withdrawn and some parentified children to be problematic. In capsulizing the four coping styles, she writes that in addition to the withdrawn child,

> parentified children can be worrisome too, because they subjugate their own needs so easily. Their behavior is similar to the pattern sometimes described as "codependency" in literature on adult children of alcoholics. Codependents don't feel like worthwhile human beings unless they are helping someone who is helpless or out of control. On the positive side, parentified children grow up to be special education teachers, pediatricians, and social workers in disproportionate numbers. On the less positive side, they get into relationships with spouses who abuse drugs or alcohol, or who are chronically unemployed—in this way they continue to have someone dysfunctional to take care of. The superachieving and mascot children probably have the healthiest adaptations because they operate with an intact sense of self that derives either from achievements outside the home or from a certain ability to view family dysfunction at a distance as reflected by their ability to use humor to describe their own difficult situations. (p. 153)

The conclusions drawn from the research on siblings is mixed (Stoneman & Berman, 1993; Seligman & Darling, 1997). Generally speaking, the impact may be "for better or for worse," depending on numerous mediating variables. I concur with Lobato's (1990) conclusion after an extensive literature review:

To many parents of young children, it may seem as though the child's illness or disability will do nothing but harm to the other children. However, this is actually quite far from the truth. As young siblings mature, evidence is clear that they usually do not have more problems than other children. In fact, many siblings show areas of great social and psychological strength. Their relationships with and behavior toward one another also tend to be more nurturing and positive than between many other sibling pairs. (p. 60)

In terms of helping siblings cope, there has been a major push to involve them in workshops and support groups designed especially for them (Meyer & Vadasy, 1994). These workshops help siblings express repressed or suppressed emotions, contribute to their knowledge about disability, and provide a social context where they can experience the company of others struggling with similar issues. Teachers should be aware of the nondisabled siblings in their classes, as they can be supportive and understanding of them, and also suggest support groups or counseling for those who may benefit from such help.

Grandparents and Other Extended Family Members

Much of the literature on families has focused on the nuclear family, with little mention of grandparents. To think of the family apart from its ancestral past is to ignore an integral aspect of the family's present life. Generally speaking, grandparents are a source of much pleasure, support, and guidance. There are exceptions, however, when grandparents are meddlesome, provide little support, and in some cases, contribute to disruption and conflict in the family. An issue that may be especially frustrating for the family is the grandparents' difficulty in grasping the seriousness of the impact of a child's disability on the family (Harris, 1994).

By their reactions and lack of support, grandparents can be a source of considerable consternation to the nuclear family coping with childhood disability. The sense of threat and vulnerability, the loss they experience, the ambiguity the situation holds for them, and their denial and lack of acceptance can indeed be burdensome for the family. In this regard, Hornby and Ashworth (1994) report that, in their small-scale study (n = 25 parents), they found that the perceived level of support from grandparents was low. One-fourth of the grandparents were considered to have added to the parents' burdens, and almost one-third of the parents expressed a wish for more support from grandparents. However, perhaps for most families of a child with special needs who have living extended family, the situation may be more positive. Indeed, as Vadasy, Fewell, and Meyer (1986) report, mothers of deaf–blind children ranked their own parents high on their list of supports.

Grandparents' contributions to the nuclear family can be many and varied. Some professionals conceive of grandparents as valuable resources to their grandchildren and the family (Vadasy et al., 1985). Due to their experience, grandparents have much to offer in advising about child care, providing access to community resources, and sharing coping strategies that helped them in the past. They also may have more time available to assist with shopping, errands, and child care; and any type of respite from the daily chores of caring for the child is welcome. Respite services are in short supply in some communities, making this a most valuable contribution. Furthermore, because of their community contacts, grandparents may be able to provide the family with access to services within the community. Through the grandparents' church group, for example, the family might gain access to child care, special equipment, and other types of support. Also, as a consequence of divorce, substance abuse, and violence, some grandparents serve as parents to children with disabilities (Simpson, 1996).

A concern of parents of infants with disabilities is whether their parents will be accepting of the baby. On the other hand, a source of consternation for grandparents who are accepting of their grandchild is how to help and be supportive of their children. They may be in a position of wanting to support the nuclear family while simultaneously grieving their own loss of a healthy grandchild. Unless there are preexisting, unresolved issues between the grandparents and the parents, these family members can be the source of considerable emotional and instrumental support. In fact, grandparents can at times be more accepting of a grandchild with a disability because they are one step removed and do not have to worry to the same extent as the parents about what the child's future will hold. However, one must not minimize the potential devastating impact a grandchild with a disability can have on the expectations of grandparents who realize the lifelong burden and reduced opportunities that this child may have for the nuclear family (Marsh, 1992).

Some grandparents have difficulty accepting their grandchild, which they may express by neglecting the parents and trivializing or denying the disability (Meyer & Vadasy, 1986). Strong negative reactions from extended family members can lead to triangulation and cut-off between and within generations (Walsh, 1989). Grandparents siding with one or the other parent can lead to triangles that harm family functioning (Pieper, 1976; Farber & Ryckman, 1965; Kahana & Kahana, 1970).

Although grandparents typically enjoyed their own parenting years, they may have looked forward to the time when the parental role would cease. The birth of a child with a disability can suddenly thrust grandparents back in time, causing them to resume a role they thought had been fulfilled:

> When my own kids were little the chaos just all seemed to go with the territory—spilled milk, scattered cereal, orange peels behind the couch, lost socks, wall-to-wall toys. I cleaned it up a dozen times a day without a second thought. Now, just bending over sometimes sparks that second thought! We don't have the peace and quiet we sometimes think we'd like to have. Sometimes I find myself thinking, "I served my time at this! What am I doing here?" (Click, 1986, p. 3)

One grandparent who was thrust into a parental role due to the parents' drug addiction remarked, "I feel I've been cheated. I'm not ready for the rocking chair, but if I want to go out with friends, I can't. I feel like something has been stolen from me" (Minkler & Roe, 1993, p. 60).

Although resentment, guilt, and anger can be destructive, such feelings must be viewed in context. Negative emotions should probably be expected and accepted, especially early on. To discourage family members from expressing their pain through anger is to encourage its expression in subtle ways; thus, major underlying issues that are never directly confronted may affect the lives of family members in more camouflaged ways. At any rate, just as professionals must understand and be accepting of the parents' anger, so, too, must they accept similar feelings from grandparents. One grandmother comments:

> Anger and hostility can be destructive forces to live with. Will anger and hostility be all this child will ever mean to me? I wondered. I suffered for him—for what he might have been, should have been. I resented what his birth had done to my lovely daughter.
>
>   I cried a lot and prayed a lot and yelled at God a lot. Then, I said, "So be it. You're sorry for yourself, but look at that child. Just look at him. Not what he might have been, but what he is. Grow up, lady." (McPhee, 1982, p. 14)

As noted earlier, grandparents are often in a position to provide both instrumental and emotional support. In working with families, providers should consider grandparents as major sources of guidance and support, and at the same time be aware that extended family members who are conflicted about the child can disrupt family functioning (Seligman, 1991; Hornby & Ashworth, 1994).

Like grandparents, aunts and uncles can also provide support and concrete help. When the relationship between sisters is good, sisters of mothers who have children with disabilities tend to provide helpful social support (Siegel, 1996). An older sister with experience raising children can be particularly helpful to the parents. Although brothers or sisters mean to be supportive, sincere attempts to be helpful can be seen as criticism, especially if the siblings are competitive with one another. Generally speaking, though, siblings with reasonably good relationships with each other can be of considerable support to the nuclear family. In conclusion, teachers and other professionals should view the extended family as an effective and generally important source of support to the nuclear family.

CHRONIC BURDEN OF CARE

The chronicity of care that families of a child with a disability anticipate is a major feature that distinguishes them from families confronting other crises that may be of a more acute and time-limited nature. For some families who have children with disabilities, the care is necessary 24 hours per day, 7 days per week, and for many years. The stresses can be relentless, draining the family physically and emotionally. Add to this the financial worries that may exist, and the family has the potential for being at risk. The degree to which the family is in trouble may depend on how its members conceptualize or reframe their life circumstance, how supportive they are of one another, and the availability of social support outside the family.

The burden of instrumental care is not only chronic, but it also may be experienced as a dark cloud that will continue to engulf the family for years to come. Family members can see little relief when they look to the future. Instead of independence, growth, and differentiation, a family may see only despair, dependence, and social isolation. The mental health needs of these parents may be cumulative; that is, living with a child with a disability over many years can take its toll psychologically, physically, and financially.

In facing the future, family members must decide how they plan to negotiate their special life circumstance. Flexibility and adaptability are important to successful family living. Without becoming intrusive, family members must be able to assume roles not ordinarily assigned by society. For example, siblings may need to help with caretaking more than they otherwise would, and fathers may need to assist instrumentally more often and also be more psychologically supportive of the mother. Mothers have to learn to facilitate, without undue guilt, as much growth and independence as their child is capable of achieving. All in all, over the family's lifespan, members need to adapt, negotiate, and communicate. This is sound advice for all families, but it has special relevance to families in which there is a chronic stressor. In families where adjustment to childhood disability is a major problem, the education professional can help by making a referral to a mental health practitioner (Laborde & Seligman, 1991).

In addition to seeking help within the family, the family system needs to be permeable enough to allow for outside help, such as respite care, when such help is needed and available. For example, Wikler (1981) reports that respite care leads to a decrease in negative maternal attitudes toward the child and increased positive family interaction. Upshur (1991) reinforces the importance of respite care services and advocates a spectrum of types of respite care to meet different family needs. Receptiveness to outside intervention and help is important in enabling the family to cope with a chronic and potentially stressful situation. And it is within this context that professional educators can help families by being accepting, empathic, open to the views of parents, and willing to make referrals to appropriate resources in the community.

DEVELOPMENTAL TRANSITIONS

Because of the nature and severity of a child's disability and the family's response to it, families of children who have disabilities must concern themselves with a series of developmental stages. Children with disabilities may be slower accomplishing certain life-cycle or developmental milestones, and some may never achieve them (Farber, 1975; Fewell, 1986). As the child approaches critical periods, parents may experience renewed anxiety or sadness (Marsh, 1992; Olshansky, 1962). Fewell (1991) describes six periods that are particularly stressful to parents of children with disabilities.

Encountering the Disability

The nature of a child's disability generally determines when the parents learn about it. Genetic disabilities, such as Down syndrome, are apparent soon after birth; therefore, parents become aware of their child's condition early. Conditions such a deafness and language and learning disabilities may not be discovered until the child is older. The confirmation of a serious and chronic problem often precipitates a crisis and affects the entire family. As noted earlier in this chapter, immediate reactions may be those of shock, great disappointment, anxiety, and depression (Hornby, 1994). The loss of the child who was expected may precipitate a mourning period much like the death of a family member. Contact with physicians and health care workers is particularly intense at this stage. It is also during this time of considerable stress that family members need to inform other family members, friends, and work acquaintances of their situation. The awkwardness some family members feel in their efforts to inform others can lead to isolation during a stressful period when social support would be very helpful. A father who found out that his daughter had Down syndrome writes:

> I didn't want to see my friends. We became very isolated as a result of it. We drifted away from a lot of friends we had—I found that I couldn't talk to friends. I couldn't face them—I think this is a little bit sad in the sense that I was very close to quite a few guys who had played soccer with me since I was very young—after Sally was born they just completely faded out of existence. (in Hornby, 1994, p. 57)

Related to the initial encounter is the notion that a child's disability is an unanticipated event. Generally speaking, adults have expectations of the normal, anticipated life-cycle events. Adults "internalize expectations of the consensually validated sequences of major life events—not only what these events should be but when they should occur" (Neugarten, 1976, p. 18). It is the unanticipated life event (e.g., birth of a child with a disability) that is likely to be experienced as a traumatic event. Major stressors tend to be caused by "off time" events that fall outside of the family's expectations (Marsh, 1992; Rolland, 1993).

Early Childhood

The early childhood years can be difficult ones for family members as they anxiously watch for their child to achieve certain developmental milestones. The chronicity of a child's disabilities and what it means to the family are a major part of the early childhood years. The nature and severity of the disability may play a key role in the family's perception and behavior (Fewell, 1991; Lyon & Lyon, 1991). In regard to a child's developmental delay, Fewell (1986) observes:

> The task of diapering a three-year-old is simply not as easy as it was when the child was one year old. The larger and heavier child requires more energy to lift and carry. The emotional burden is also great: parents anticipate the end of diapers and two o'clock bottles, and when these things don't end, it can shatter dreams and invite questions about the future. (pp. 16–17)

Concerns about what the future holds for the child and family begin to emerge during early childhood and for some, as early as infancy. One parent's concern about the future is vividly portrayed by educator and parent Helen Featherstone (1980):

> I remember, during the early months of Jody's life, the anguish with which I contemplated the distant future. Jody cried constantly, not irritable, hungry cries, but heartrending shrieks of pain. Vain efforts to comfort him filled my nights and days. One evening when nothing seemed to help, I went outside, intending to escape his misery for a moment, hoping that without me he might finally fall asleep. Walking in summer darkness, I imagined myself at seventy, bent and wrinkled, hobbling up the stairs to minister to Jody, now over forty, but still crying and helpless. (p. 19)

Although early intervention programs are generally applauded, a crisis may develop when a child enters an early intervention program, because of the following:

1. Families see older children with a similar condition and wonder whether their child will resemble them as he or she develops.
2. Families who share their experiences with other families realize that they may need to "fight" for the services their child needs, further draining the families' resources.
3. Families learn that they are often expected to be their child's primary caregivers and teachers. In this regard, Turnbull and Turnbull (1986) quote a mother who says, "I found the infant stimulation program to be very helpful in providing an opportunity to learn parenting skills. (Peter was our first child.) It also helped our morale in that it gave us specific things to teach

Peter, so we could see steady progress in his development. This created strong feelings of guilt in me because I felt that if I wasn't working with him at every opportunity, then I wasn't doing enough. If his progress was slow, I felt it was my fault" (p. 51).

During this phase, parents come into increasingly more contact with professionals who may treat parents as patients who need treatment rather than as expert parents and caregivers (Seligman & Seligman, 1980; Alper et al., 1994). Perhaps most discouraging at this stage is the realization of the chronic burden a child might be for the family as they view the future with some degree of uncertainty and anxiety. However, early intervention programs help to prepare the family for the marathon ahead.

School Entry

Parents may experience another setback or period of adjustment when they realize that their child fails to fit into the mainstream of the traditional education system (Marshak et al., 1999). A child may require special education classes and a separate transportation system. Siblings may find this a particularly difficult period, as more of their schoolmates learn that they have a brother or sister who has a disability. This stage can be characterized as the period when the family members "go public," as they venture beyond the boundaries of the family. Also, if they have not done so already, parents must adjust the educational and vocational goals they had envisioned for their child. However, parents should be reassured that as some doors are closed to their children, others will open.

It is important to note again that the difficulties parents experience depend on the nature of the child's disability (e.g., there may be relatively few adjustments if the child is moderately physically disabled) and the preparedness of the school system to provide adequate educational and adjunct services for children with special needs. Also, during this period, parents may debate the merits of a segregated versus inclusive educational setting for their child.

Adolescence

Adolescence marks the period when children begin to separate from their parents. This period also reflects the time when adolescent children experience considerable change, turmoil, and ambivalence. For families of children with disabilities, this stage can be a painful reminder of their children's failure to successfully traverse this life-cycle stage as they continue to remain dependent (Marshak et al., 1999).

Peer acceptance, or the lack of it, may be particularly painful for the entire family during the adolescent years. Peer acceptance may determine the extent to which the child experiences rejection and isolation, which in turn may contribute to the stress parents and siblings experience. The issues of deviance and conformity are particularly salient during the adolescent years. In a book chapter, I expressed concerns about my children's experience of rejection thusly:

> As Lori grew to pre-adolescence and adolescence her deficiencies became more obvious and the adulation she basked in earlier was replaced by a certain amount of scorn and rejection. The kids congregating in the neighborhood cul-de-sac played with her only if others were unavailable. Although a few of the neighborhood children seemed to be fond of her, I was aware that some children chronically taunted her and referred to her as "slow" and a "retard." As Lori's sib, Lisa had to make instantaneous decisions about whether she was going to side with her sister or the neighborhood kids. If she sided with her sister, Lisa jeopardized her friendship with the other kids and, if she supported Lori, I wondered whether she was angry at her pals and angry toward Lori for being different and threatening her friendships. This must have been an insufferable bind. I often observed the kids interacting from our living room window. My heart ached to see either Lisa or Lori hurt. I felt impotent to help either one avoid the pain. (Seligman, 1995, pp. 175–176)

Because of their disabilities, adolescents deviate from their non-disabled peers. The issues of deviance and conformity are particularly salient during the adolescent years.

> Adolescence is a particularly difficult phase of life for many with disabilities. The value placed on conformity during adolescence typically causes considerable distress because of the difference inherent in having a disability. Differentness becomes bad. An additional source of distress is the heightened importance placed on attracting a member of the opposite sex. Issues of independence and emancipation also become pronounced and a source of considerable turmoil. (Marshak & Seligman, 1993, p. 14)

Beginning Adult Life

Public education offers both children and parents several benefits. It helps the child gain important educational and vocational skills, independence, and provides respite for the parents. But as a child's education draws to an end, parents must make some difficult choices. Because of limited vocational possibilities and inadequate community living arrangements, some families may be left with few choices. This is a stressful period in that the specter of the child's future looms and can cause considerable concern and anxiety. A thorough discussion of this phase appears in the book *Disability and the Family Life Cycle* by Marshak et al. (1999).

Maintaining Adult Life

Where an adult with a disability will live and the level of care characterize the family's concerns at this stage. A major concern is the future care of their adult child as parents worry about the ensuing years, when they may not be able to be active overseers, or when they are deceased. I wrote about my fears regarding my young adult daughter when I am no longer alive: "Tears come to my eyes when I think of Lori without her parents. She is so accustomed to having them around. I try to suppress the apprehension that wells up in me when thoughts of Lori's future come to mind. But I can't deny the reality that anxieties about Lori's future are relentless" (Seligman, 1995, p. 182).

At this time, mental health professionals are particularly important to help families plan for their child's future in terms of vocational and leisure-time activities, and in terms of living arrangements. Attorneys and other experts in the area of future and estate planning can be helpful during this stage as well. Adult siblings, as well as other extended family members, may be a useful resource and should be explored as potential helpers during this period. Although community support services are always needed, their availability and accessibility become particularly acute here. In a fitting conclusion to her discussion of the aforementioned stages, Fewell (1986) notes:

> When a family has a disabled child, all the actors in this support network must adapt to the extended needs of the disabled member. The adaptations family members make are often significant, and individual destinies may be determined by the experience. Family adaptations change as the child matures; the stress at various periods may af-

fect family members differently, for much depends on the familial and environmental contributions to the dynamic interactions of adaptation at a given point in time. (p. 19)

This chapter has explored the numerous issues with which families must contend as they attempt to construct a gratifying life with their child who has a disability. These aspects of family dynamics are critical for teachers and other school officials to be aware of as they interact with these families. The next chapter addresses issues that pertain to successful conferencing.

5

Basic Principles
of Interviewing

By now, the reader is aware of the reasons parent–teacher conferences are necessary and why they often include but also go beyond the communication of a child's academic progress. Conferences are generally initiated by teachers, but parents, the school social worker, the school nurse, a counselor, or the school psychologist may also request them. The notion that teachers may be considerably less effective conducting parent conferences than when they are teaching children is a very real possibility that must be faced by educators as well as the training institutions responsible for their education.

We are now ready to consider building relationships and developing facilitative interpersonal skills. It is important to remember that the attitudes and actual interpersonal dimensions included in this chapter are designed to increase educator's facilitative skills and not to prepare them to become counselors or psychotherapists. In other words, attitudes such as being nonjudgmental and accepting, as well as such skills as listening attentively, using questions appropriately, being supportive, and the like, are emphasized in this chapter as opposed to the acquisition of in-depth psychotherapeutic skills.

PERSONALITY CHARACTERISTICS
AND INTERPERSONAL STYLE

Even though this chapter and Chapter 6 focus on skills that may seem somewhat foreign to teachers, it is generally a good idea to practice them and try to assess the degree of "fit" between that behavior and one's personality. Teachers may wish to monitor how comfortable the new behavior or skill appears to be. Before discarding a behavior that seems unnatural, teachers should try to integrate it into their natural style of response. It would be unusual if the new behavior did not feel somewhat awkward; many new experiences do.

A word of caution is in order. I embrace the point of view that new behaviors should be at least minimally compatible with a person's natural style of response. In other words, new behaviors or skills should be incorporated into one's natural way of interacting with others. It is the newly learned behavior that is subject to modification, not one's characteristic style of response. For example, teachers are encouraged to engage others with a considerable amount of eye contact; but if a teacher happens to be a sensitive and perceptive listener with a lesser degree of eye contact, insisting on a change in this behavior would be contraindicated. In such an instance, the teacher would give other assurances of interest and attention through an accurate verbal response to indicate that he or she is listening.

VALUES AND THE
PARENT–TEACHER CONFERENCE

Having lived for a particular span of time during which we have encountered many people, experiences, and beliefs, we inevitably develop values about many aspects of life. Some values involve preferences in food, automobiles, clothes, schools, flowers, movies, politics, music, and so on. Differences of opinion between individuals over these preferences (or values) might take the form of a friendly discussion about the virtues of Beethoven's music over that of Mozart, or opinions as to who is the greatest all-around baseball player of all time.

Other values can lead to powerful emotions, to strong and sometimes inflexible convictions that may contribute to strained interpersonal communication and, under certain circumstances, may even polarize large groups of people. Such values, for example, are concerned with issues related to religion, politics, abortion, integration, and sexual behavior and orientation.

Of course, all of us have values. We might consider parent–teacher conferences as encounters of two unique sets of values. Strong feelings about religion or politics, for example, are generally not discussed in a parent–teacher conference, yet they are not *always* absent. Parents may communicate strong convictions, perhaps related to their child's disability or about abortion, that run counter to those of the teacher. Or parents may openly support a candidate for election who is opposed to pay raises for teachers. In such instances, the teacher must remember the purpose of the conference, namely, to help the parents, to communicate observations of their child, and so on. A heated discussion over religious or political views has no place in a parent–teacher conference.

What I am suggesting is that the teacher adopt a philosophy of neutrality. She may respond with anger or resentment, and her stomach may feel knotted, or her palms may be perspiring, but she is aware of what is happening internally *and why* is important. The notion that parents have as much right to their point of view as the teacher is a reality that requires a considerable degree of acceptance. Parental values do not have to be synonymous with those of the teacher to have effective conferences.

The more we know about our own values and how they evolved, the more accepting we can be of the values of others. Such self-enlightenment helps set the stage for a productive, tension-free meeting. Benjamin (1987) believes that by not judging others' values, professionals create a comfortable environment:

> Basically, to me acceptance means treating the interviewee [parent] as an equal and regarding his thoughts and feelings with sincere respect. It does not mean agreeing; it does not mean thinking or feeling the way he does; it does not mean valuing what he values. It is, rather the attitude that the interviewee [parent] has as much right to his ideas, feelings, and values as I have to mine and that I want to do my utmost to understand his life space in terms of his ideas, feelings, and values rather than in terms of my own. Such an attitude is difficult to maintain and even more difficult to communicate to the interviewee. At times it may be misunderstood, interpreted as agreement, consent, or reassurance. And yet we have no choice but to attempt to be accepting. Otherwise, the interviewee will suspect that we are judging him, asking him to feel and think as we do or, even worse, to think and feel as we believe he ought to be thinking and feeling. (p. 39)

Values that are important for social workers and psychologists are equally relevant for teachers who conduct parent conferences: "Clinical interviews should reflect that clinicians value the dignity and worth of all people. Clinicians [teachers] should convey a nonjudgmental acceptance without necessarily approving of specific behaviors. Clinicians [teachers] should actively work toward eliminating ways of thinking, speaking, and acting that reflect racism, sexism, ableism, ageism, homophobia, religious discrimination, and other oppressive ideologies" (Murphy & Dillon, 1998, p. 10).

The following exercise developed by Schulman (1978, pp. 53–54) will help readers become aware of their values: Make a list of the behavioral traits in people that annoy you. Then rate the items on a scale from 1 to 5 (rate the most bothersome items 5, the least bothersome, 1). Gather all your 5 ratings and all your 1 ratings and study them carefully. What do these lists tell you about yourself?

Now, we turn to an examination of values held by the teacher. It is not unusual to find ourselves in a position of dissuading a friend or relative of a particular point of view—and this is to be anticipated and accepted in a social encounter in which there is little or no disparity in status. In a conference with a parent, however, the imposition of a teacher's values should be most assiduously avoided: "The hazard lies in an imposition of values by the counselor [teacher]. The danger is great because the counselor may not consciously intend for this to happen. But when it does happen, the counselee [parent] feels somewhat pushed down as a person. An implied denial of the worth of his own views and experiences is given to him, and he senses the disapproval and rejection of himself as he is at the moment" (Johnson & Vestermark, 1970, p. 78).

Ross (1964), who wrote the pioneering book *The Exceptional Child in the Family*, is adamant about the view that "the professional must . . . attempt an honest examination of his own feelings and attitudes before he can expect to be helpful and if he is unable to do so, he will need a consultant, supervisor, or therapist who can help him with this examination" (p. 73).

We know from previous chapters that professionals are often less objective about families whose backgrounds are either greatly different from their own or so similar as to recall attitudes and feelings from which they may wish to disassociate. Should such unconsciously (or perhaps even consciously) held beliefs exist, the teacher may assess parents inaccurately, be unable to surmount communication barriers imposed by different social histories, or make inappropriate or poor judgments about parental strengths or weaknesses. Thus, teachers must be aware of prejudices and blind spots and work hard at overcoming them, or, at the very least, keep them in their proper perspective during conferences.

THE SETTING OF THE CONFERENCE

The physical setting of the interview is largely a matter of personal preference. If possible, the conference should be held in a room where there are no external distractions and where the participants may not be overheard. Most teachers do not have an office available to them, so the use of their classrooms should suffice if these conditions are met.

Murphy and Dillon (1998) agree that the environment of a conference should be free of distractions and private, so that conversations are confidential. These authors also believe that the physical environment should be accessible to persons with disabilities and flexible enough to allow for comfortable personal space. "Most people have an invisible area around them that serves as a protective barrier. Intrusion into this personal space creates discomfort. Personal space varies from person to person, culture to culture, and situation to situation" (p. 23).

These authors also note that gender plays a role in personal space preferences in that in Western cultures, men create more space between themselves and male strangers than do women with female strangers. Typically, North Americans prefer a talking space of about an arm's length, the British tend to want more space, Hispanic people prefer even less distance, and people from the Middle East can converse practically eyeball to eyeball (Ivey, 1994, cited in Murphy & Dillon, 1998). Personal space can also be influenced by issues related to position and power. Typically, persons with less power have their personal space imposed upon by those with greater power. Given these different space requirements, it would be prudent for teachers to have movable chairs when they confer with parents, so that they may accommodate a variety of circumstances.

Sitting behind a large desk is often viewed negatively, since physical objects of any size are felt to represent barriers to a comfortable interpersonal exchange. To some extent, this is a matter of choice and comfort. Some teachers, especially when they are novices, feel more comfortable having a physical object between themselves and the parent. In this case, sitting in one's chair behind a desk in the following fashion:

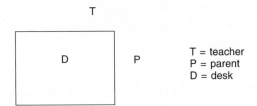

is considerably more desirable than the following alternative:

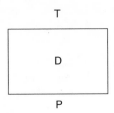

The most desirable seating arrangement for an interview is to place two comfortable chairs reasonably close to each other, at a 90-degree angle, with a small table nearby.

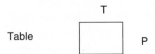

This arrangement allows parents to look at the teacher or straight ahead, whichever makes them feel more comfortable at any particular point in the conference. It also allows the teacher to vary her gaze, depending on her comfort or that of the parent. Cups for coffee or glasses for soft drinks may be placed on the small table for the convenience of either party.

It is unwise to have parents wait much beyond their scheduled appointment, an action that implicitly conveys a lack of interest, respect, and concern. In addition to being an inconvenience, a protracted wait may be considered rude and generate feelings of frustration and anger that can get the conference participants off on the wrong foot.

As noted previously, there should be no noise and distractions of any sort (Kroth & Edge, 1997). Those who wish to discuss important matters with a professional want that person's undivided attention. The following interruptions can only hinder the conference: phone calls, people who want "just a word with you," secretaries who must have something signed immediately, and so on. Arrangements should be made to complete any administrative details prior to the conference, and secretaries and others who might inadvertently "pop in" should be advised that you will be occupied for a specified period of time. Some enterprising teachers hang "Do Not Disturb" signs on the conference-room door. Furthermore, conferences are best held when all or most children and other school personnel have left for the day. Ensuring that the conversation between the teacher and parent is held in privacy is important in developing trust and good feelings. The need for privacy and confidentiality is so important that it bears repeating.

It is sometimes helpful to make a few notes about certain parental concerns or to jot down some information or data about the child. However, continuous or even frequent note taking *during* a conference is to be avoided unless it is *essential*. Continuous note taking is often considered rude, but it also conveys a sense of disinterest and over-concern with details and cold facts. To keep brief records of parent conferences the teacher, at her leisure, can jot down the gist of the conference for future reference or for school record purposes *after* the parent leaves. Continuous note taking during a conference may be indicative of the teacher's attempt to maintain distance or to calm herself from the intensity of a parent–teacher meeting.

Finally, the possibility of having a conference at the parents' home should not be ruled out, especially when meetings at the school may be a hardship for parents (Hornby, 1995; Berger, 1981). Indeed, Shea and Bauer (1991) report that home visits by teachers are increasingly common and may be an expected part of their job. School administrators and school boards are demonstrating greater willingness to be more flexible and adjust school schedules to accommodate home visits. The rationale for home visits is articulated by Shea and Bauer (1991):

> A home visit helps the teacher get to know the child's family, environment, and culture better in order to serve both child and parents more effectively. A conference at home is an occasion for the teacher to meet the other members of the child's educational team and become acquainted with the child's learning context. Teachers can use home visits for several purposes: information gathering, reporting the child's school performance, problem solving, preliminary discussions for the formal IEP meeting, and parent training.

Because the home conference takes place in the child's natural environment, the teacher's careful observation can often answer questions about the child's behavior and academic achievement, particularly the quality of the interactions between the child and other people in the household. In the home setting, the teacher can express concerns about the child directly in a face-to-face discussion: because the parents are in a familiar and secure environment during the home conference, they are more willing to express concerns about the child, teacher, and school. (p. 159)

Such a conference can give the teacher a more complete picture of the child's environment. It also reinforces the positive perception of the teacher's interest and concern in that she may be seen as extending herself beyond the call of duty. Home visits are also desirable because they allow working parents and/or both parents the opportunity to confer with the teacher. In considering a conference in the parents' home, the teacher should be sensitive to the parent who might feel that such a visit would be an imposition or an indication of the teacher's nosiness.

Whether at school or at home, early meetings (either before the school year begins or shortly thereafter) with parents tend to diminish problems of attendance, discipline, and dropouts, and have a favorable effect on grades and subsequent home and school conferences (Duncan & Fitzgerald, 1969, cited in Seligman, 1979). Hornby (1995) and Shea and Bauer (1991) offer the following guidelines for home visits: Home visits should always be prearranged. Never make unannounced visits to a child's home. Hornby (1995) advises that since parents will be dressed casually, teachers should dress less formally also to help parents feel at ease. The purpose of the conference should never be a mystery and should be communicated well before the home visit. Ambiguity about the purpose of the meeting is discourteous and increases anxiety. Parents should know how long a meeting will last so that they can plan postmeeting activities, such as dinner preparations. In terms of time, it is important for teachers to be punctual.

At the beginning of the visit, teachers can talk informally for a brief period of time to set a friendly and relaxed tone. Teachers should keep in mind that such visits are not inspection tours. They are guests who want to avoid judging interactions and conditions in the home. At the same time, they observe and assess interactions that will ultimately benefit the child and his parents (Shea & Bauer, 1991). Also, keep in mind that cultural factors may determine the teacher's behavior:

"When I was teaching in New Zealand and made a home visit to a Samoan family I found that they had prepared a full meal of Samoan food all served on banana leaves for my arrival. Fortunately, I had been forewarned that it is not possible to discuss important matter in a Samoan household until you have eaten with the family" (Hornby, 1995, pp. 110–111).

In contrast to visits at school, teachers should anticipate that there are likely to be distractions during a home visit. In their discussion of home visits, Shea and Bauer (1991) conclude that "home visits do have disadvantages. They are time-consuming and often inconvenient for both parents and teachers. Both parties must prepare for the visit. However, the many advantages of meeting on the child's home ground generally outweigh the disadvantages" (p. 161).

ESTABLISHMENT OF GOALS

Toward the beginning of the first teacher–parent meeting, the teacher may wish to consider how he might facilitate movement toward shared goals. Conferences normally begin with a certain amount of small talk about the weather, inflation, or an event in the news. This conversation is to be expected and serves the function of warming up and settling in before pursuing serious business. Abrupt, discourteous interruptions of this kind of talk are to be discouraged. For example, it would be inappropriate, after a short period of time, for the teacher to comment, "I know you didn't come here to talk about the kidnapping of Karen Green so let's get down to business." Sooner or later, one of the two participants will gradually begin to discuss the anticipated content of the meeting. People tend to sense when the time has arrived to begin to address more serious concerns. An abrupt response generally signals feelings of nervousness and impatience or, more seriously, indicates an insensitive teacher. Generally, both teachers and parents have agreed to a specific period of time to meet, so this should help set the pace of the conference. By the way, *both* parents and teachers should know when the meeting begins and ends *before* the actual conference.

Whatever the objectives of a conference, it is important to keep the following principles in mind:

1. Working objectives should be clear.
2. Objectives should be mutually agreed upon.

3. There should be a timetable established for their accomplishment.
4. Goals should indicate the expected outcome.
5. Goals should be realistic.
6. Goals should be attainable. (Heaton, 1998, pp. 87–88)

When unanticipated topics arise, the most productive posture is to remain calm, expect surprises, and try not to explain them away or become defensive. The conference goal may shift from what the teacher had set initially to one of thoughtful listening, understanding, and responding. Interpersonal interactions are not programmed mechanical meetings, where the content and outcome is always predictable. What Lisbe (1978) noted over 20 years ago still holds true today: "The realities of 'people work' require a presence unlike other fields where processes are replicable. Carpenters follow blue prints, automobile manufacturers use molds, accountants work from forms, and pilots read instrument panels. There are no such guidelines when one human being faces another, where the uniqueness of each encounter requires uncompromising intensity" (p. 242).

During the course of a conference with a general goal (e.g., the biyearly parent–teacher conference about a child's performance at school), the parents may mention, for example, that they are in the midst of divorce proceedings that may have implications for the child's future. Generally, such an event is communicated to alert the teacher to anticipated changes in the child's environment that may affect his schoolwork, his emotions, and behavior. Possibly, the disclosure also serves a cathartic purpose; that is, it provides the parents with a chance to talk about an impending, emotion-filled event. In either case, empathic and supportive listening is all that is called for in most instances of this nature. Teachers should know that parents in difficult situations, often bombarded with well-intentioned but mostly unnecessary advice from a variety of sources, welcome the presence of an interested listener.

Another example is when a parent calls in an obvious state of distress and requests a conference without disclosing the problem. This type of call may be disquieting to a teacher, who begins to search for the possible cause of the parent's concern, sometimes feeling that he has engaged in some sort of indiscretion. However, in this type of situation, clear-cut anticipated goals must be abandoned, except for one: careful, sensitive, attentive listening and appropriate responding.

Schulman (1978) discusses three general types of goal-oriented interviews, two of which are relevant to this discussion and, thus, are examined here.

THE INFORMATION-ORIENTED INTERVIEW

The information-oriented interview is not designed to deepen the contact between people but instead focuses on the collection of information or data. Some examples are public opinion polls, personnel interviews, or journalistic interviews.

Both the parent and teacher may, at different times during their relationship, need to seek information from each other. For example, the teacher may wish to gently probe the various facets of the child's home environment. Generally, questions about a child's family situation need not be asked directly. Over a period of time, the teacher gradually becomes aware of the family configuration, the feelings the parent as well as the siblings have toward the child with a disability, and the available support system. Gathering information is a gradual and ongoing process that takes place over time.

Parents may need information that they can ask for quite directly. In responding to questions, the teacher should try to be open; when asked a personal question or one she does not wish to answer for some reason, she should politely decline to give a full response. It is unlikely that a teacher will be asked a very personal question. More likely, information-seeking questions such as the following may be anticipated: "How long have you been teaching at this school?" "Have you worked with children who are retarded long?" "Can you tell me how Adam is doing in his arithmetic?" "How have the other children been interacting with Adam?" "Have you lived in this town for many years or are you a newcomer?" "From which college did you get your education?"

Sometimes, a parent asks questions like these just to make small talk, or so that the parent will feel on an equal footing with the teacher. Other parents may ask semipersonal questions to form an impression of the teacher. One question may relate to whether the teacher has had personal experiences with disability, for example, "Are you a parent of a child with disabilities?" Such questions should be answered honestly and without rancor. As noted, questions are often asked to establish a relationship and to see whether the participants have had similar experiences, although people can look to others for common experiences. During initial meetings in social situations, human beings collect data on each other so that they can decide about developing potential friendships based on similarities in values and interests.

Social psychologists have explored and written extensively on how variables in interpersonal attraction play an important role in the maintenance of friendships (Berscheid & Walster, 1969; Rubin, 1973; Napier & Gershenfeld, 1999). Although the parent–teacher encounter resembles a professional rather than a personal relationship, and therefore some of the variables in interpersonal attraction are less salient than other factors in determining the course of the relationship, nevertheless, some sizing up of one another does take place.

During professional meetings—and to some extent in more personal encounters also—initial impressions are either reinforced, modified, or completely discarded as the relationship continues. The teacher may feel that some evaluative processes are in motion during initial conferences. In fact, it is not unusual for initial meetings between two people to be exploratory and to some extent superficial. Information-oriented interviews, then, serve a definite and important socializing and sizing-up purpose.

THE EXPERIENTIAL INTERVIEW

The experiential interview *focuses on the relationship* between the parties. Sharing thoughts and feelings within an accepting atmosphere is the hallmark of this interview. Judgmental attitudes have no place here. "This kind of interview becomes a microunit of life in which two people, the interviewer and interviewee, share feelings, understandings and behavior—a small unit of life experience in which the individuals involved share themselves" (Schulman, 1978, p. 78). An illustration of an experiential interview follows. (Johnny's mother is distressed over his lack of progress in school and has a conference with the teacher to discuss her concerns.)

TEACHER: Hello, Mrs. Wright. I'm glad we have a chance to get together. Would you care to sit down? [A welcoming remark.]

MRS. WRIGHT: Thank you. I feel foolish coming here to talk to you about this when I know you have other things to do.

TEACHER: It sounds as if you do not wish to intrude on my time and that your concerns about Johnny seem minor compared to my other activities. I can understand how you feel, but I believe it is important to meet with the parents of the children I teach. The fact that *you* feel that we should get together tells me that our meeting is important. [The teacher is reflecting what she believes the parent is feeling, empathizing with her and assuaging her feelings of guilt and insignificance.]

MRS. WRIGHT: Well, I do feel somewhat better about taking up your time. I've come to talk to you about what my husband and I see as a lack of progress on Johnny's part. [Feeling less of an intruder now and sensing that the teacher is attentive, she proceeds.]

TEACHER: I wonder if you could be a bit more specific. Are you referring to his progress academically or are you referring to his behavior? [To be able to respond adequately, the teacher requests additional information.]

MRS. WRIGHT: I am referring to his schoolwork. As a matter of fact, Johnny has become much more manageable at home than he has been. In contrast to the past, he is actually a pleasure to live with. That is one of the reasons why we don't want to say too much about the drop in his academic subjects.

TEACHER: It sounds as if you are pleased with the progress Johnny is making in his behavior but are concerned that if you mention his schoolwork he may not be as pleasant to live with. [The teacher is correctly *ferreting out and communicating* the crux of the problem.]

MRS. WRIGHT: That's exactly right. My husband and I are afraid that he may become uncontrollable again if we push his schoolwork. We are very much concerned about this and are not quite sure whether we should leave him alone or push his schoolwork. [Implicitly asking for advice from the teacher.]

TEACHER: I can see the quandary you're in. You want Johnny to continue his social progress but you also don't want him to ignore schoolwork. Let me describe what has been happening with Johnny at school and perhaps some way of dealing with the situation will become clear. I agree with your observations that Johnny is paying less attention to schoolwork. But I've noticed that he has been making a strong effort to develop friendships with others in class. As a matter of fact, his efforts are beginning to pay off. He has developed a relationship with two people in class—relationships that I see becoming stronger over time. Along with these friendships has come a greater acceptance of Johnny on the part of others in the class. My guess is that Johnny is learning that when he gives others a chance, he can develop friendships and that he really is a likable person. He seems to be getting positive attention from others by being kind and reaching out rather than by being mean and abusive. It seems that his newly discovered social life is so demanding that he puts all his effort into his relationships at school *and* at home and that his schoolwork is slipping. I can't say for sure, but my guess is that as less energy is concentrated in becoming an acceptable friend and a welcome family member, he will begin to consider more seriously his academic status. What do you think about my hypothesis? [The teacher provides observations and *ventures* a hypothesis that may lead the parent to a course of action. The teacher is also asking for the parent's input.]

MRS. WRIGHT: What you are saying is that making friends with others seems to be very important to him now and that when he feels more comfortable with others his attention will hopefully shift to his schoolwork. If that's so, I think that it might be a good idea to continue to work on *our* relationship with him at home and lay off the academics for the time being. [The parent is led to a conclusion with the guidance of the teacher, who quickly comprehended her concern, empathized with her feelings, provided her with data from observations at school, and presented a way, without lecturing or giving direct advice, in which she could deal with the child. This method allows the parent to arrive at her own conclusions, based on a better understanding of the problem and by possessing the data required to take action.]

TEACHER: What you are saying makes a lot of sense to me. I'll try to do the same at school. Why don't we talk again in another 2 months to see how things are going? Should we set up a meeting time now? [The teacher reinforces the idea that the parent made the decision about how to proceed, and she offers to meet again to reevaluate the situation.]

In contrast to the information-oriented interview, the experiential interview may include information or data, but stress is placed on the feelings behind expressed verbalizations, accurately comprehending the problem by reflecting the content of the interview, sharing perceptions with the parent, being supportive, and facilitating the decision- or resolution-making process for the parent.

LISTENING

The reader may question the wisdom of including a section on listening. Most of us assume that we all listen and that we listen well. Take a few moments to reflect on situations where someone else was physically present, ostensibly hearing what you were saying and yet not really *listening* to what you were trying to convey. All of us have encountered parents, friends, teachers, and supervisors who hear but do not listen. More often than not, our reaction to this inattention is to feel hurt, ignored, or angry.

In his book, *The Lost Art of Listening*, Nichols (1995) offers his view of listening as a way of connecting with others:

> The yearning to be listened to and understood is a yearning to escape our separateness and bridge the space that divides us. We reach out and try to overcome that separateness by revealing what's on our minds and in our hearts, hoping for understanding. Getting that understanding should be simple, but it isn't.
>
> The essence of good listening is empathy, which can be achieved only by suspending our preoccupation with ourselves and entering into the experience of the other person. Part intuition and part effort, it's the stuff of human connection.
>
> A listener's empathy—understanding what we're trying to say and showing it—builds a bond of understanding, linking us to someone who understands and cares and thus confirming that our feelings are recognizable and legitimate. The power of empathic listening is the power to transform relationships. When deeply felt but unexpressed feelings take shape in words that are shared and come back clarified, the result is a reassuring sense of being understood and a grateful feeling of shared humanness with the one who understands.
>
> If listening strengthens our relationships by cementing our connection with one another, it also fortifies our sense of self. In the presence of a receptive listener, we're able to clarify what we think and discover what we feel. Thus, in giving an account of our experience to someone who listens, we are better able to listen to ourselves. Our lives are co-authored in dialogue. (p. 10)

Nothing hurts more than the sense that people close to us aren't really listening to what we have to say. We never outgrow the need to communicate what it feels like to live in our separate, private worlds of experience. That's why a sympathetic ear is such a powerful force in hu-

man relationships—and why the failure to be heard and understood is
so painful. (p. 1)

Frequently, the reaction to a nonlistener is to change the subject,
physically remove oneself from the situation, or uncomfortably continue on with the fragmented and superficial chatter. When sufficiently angered, we sometimes "return the favor" by in turn becoming
inattentive ourselves.

What are some of the characteristics of good listeners? What behaviors are involved? What are some of the indicators of a poor listener? What specific skills can one develop to become a better listener?
These are some of the questions addressed in this section.

Listening is not a mechanical activity. It is hard work and requires
deep concentration and patience, yet it becomes easier with practice. It
involves hearing the way things are being said, the tone used, while
observing the speaker's gestures. In listening attentively, one must
hear what is not said, what is hinted at, what may be held back, or
what lies beneath the surface. We must learn to listen with our third
ear (Reik, 1972), or to put it more concretely, we hear with our ears, but
we listen with our eyes and mind and heart and skin and guts as well
(Ekman, 1964).

Benjamin (1987) proposes a simple test to determine whether one
is learning to listen: "If during the interview you can state in your own
words what the interviewee has said and also convey to him in your
own words the feelings he has expressed and he then accepts all this as
emanating from him, there is an excellent chance that you have lis-
tened and understood him" (p. 45). There is no need to wait for a parent meeting to practice Benjamin's suggestion. It can be tried with
friends, relatives, or colleagues.

The interviewer should be as physically relaxed as possible, so
that careful listening is accomplished more easily. This step is so important to good listening that one may want to take a deep breath four
or five times to ease tension before a conference, or find another
method to relax so that one feels physically at ease.

Kroth and Edge (1997) present a conceptualization of the phenomenon of listening by constructing the following model on the next page.

Quadrant *A*: Passive Listener

The passive listener is "there." He is with the parent in the present. In
effect, he thinks out loud with the parent, conveying the feeling that

A Listening Paradigm

Listening

```
      A │ B
Passive ─┼─ Active
      C │ D
```

Nonlistening

what is being said is indeed understood. Nonverbal signs of acceptance—leaning forward, slight head nods, a smile—assure the parent that it is all right to continue to talk. Another term used to describe the passive listener, and one that has a more positive connotation, is "supportive listener." Often, the parent is surprised that he could talk so much in the teacher's presence or that so much time could have passed. Hornby (1995) tells a story about the power of listening and how it is often dismissed as an unhelpful activity:

> While in Bangalore a few years ago, I was told a story that I have heard many times before but which bears retelling because its message is so important. A parent who has a daughter who is mentally handicapped told me how a young mother whose child had just been diagnosed with a disability had come to him for help. They had talked for over two hours but my friend felt frustrated because he was not able to provide any practical help for the mother. He felt particularly inadequate because in India, as in many other traditional cultures, people who seek help expect to be given specific advice to follow. Therefore, it was much to his surprise when, two weeks later, the young mother called in to see my friend to thank him for all the help he had given her when they last met! He was surprised because all he had done had been to listen with understanding to what his fellow parent had to say. (p. 87)

Quadrant *B*: Active Listener

Kroth and Edge (1997) characterize the active listener as one who leans forward and maintains more than the usual amount of eye contact during a meeting. Verbally important and complex statements are reflected back to the parent (e.g., "What you seem to be telling me is that you are worried about Sam's inability to make friends and his increasing isolation. Is that pretty much what is concerning you?"). Such comments by teachers are designed to check the accuracy of their perceptions. During the conference, it is important that teachers not dominate the interview by talking more than the parent, nor should they engage in moralizing. The basic goal is to listen carefully and then respond appropriately by clarifying the issues and helping the parent to put it in perspective. You want the parent to feel understood, because by not feeling understood by the teacher, the parent will question the teacher's ability to be attentive and caring, and he may even question the teacher's competence. Hornby (1995) believes that when teachers are first learning how to listen actively, they might consider using a formula that is characterized by the words "You feel _____ because. . . . " For example, a teacher might say the following to a parent: "*You feel* disappointed *because* your husband wasn't able to come to the conference with you today" or, in a slight variation, "You seem to be feeling 'down in the dumps' today because you're not happy with Tim's report card."

Quadrant *C*: Passive Nonlistener

This type of listener simply does not concentrate on what is being said. Not only is content ignored or misunderstood but also underlying feelings are bypassed. To the parent, this is a most frustrating interpersonal encounter. Passive nonlisteners who are partially attentive may pick up some content, miss the rest, and be completely ignorant of affect (emotions).

A teacher may be particularly prone to passive nonlistening when a number of parent–teacher conferences have been held in succession. In such instances, the teacher must make a concerted effort to block out previous conferences and overcome fatigue to listen attentively to the parent in front of her. Perhaps a more sensible plan would be to space conferences over a couple of days, or at least to build in some breathing time by taking breaks between conferences.

As one approaches the end of a difficult day and begins to reflect on what has occurred, it is very easy to slip into passive nonlistening. We should all be allowed these temporary transgressions. Only if passive nonlistening begins to become a pattern does the matter become serious.

Quadrant *D*: Active Nonlistener

Social chatter at a party is an example of active nonlistening. In such instances, people talk to or *at* each other but seldom *with* each other.

Neither party is particularly interested in what the other has to say, and their conversations are fragmented; that is, what person *a* says is not picked up by person *b*, who will normally introduce another topic. In conferences where both the parent and teacher have separate agendas, the possibility of such a fragmented exchange is greatly increased:

TEACHER: I'm so glad you could come. I've been wanting to talk with you about Billy.

PARENT: I'm having trouble getting Billy to do his homework. He always wants to put it off, and we have frightful arguments about this at home.

TEACHER: He's been fighting on the playground. I've had to keep him in from recess twice this week.

PARENT: I don't think he understands the new math. That's probably why he doesn't do his homework. I wish you could do something about it.

TEACHER: Do you have any idea why he's started fighting so much? Does he ever talk about it at home? We just don't know what to do with him. It's getting to be a real problem.

PARENT: We're having a real problem, too. We're open for any suggestions. This arguing that Billy does is getting both of us upset.

TEACHER: We at school want to cooperate in any way that we can. If you have any ideas about his fighting, call me, will you? It's sure been nice taking to you, and I'm so glad you could come. You're always welcome at school.

PARENT: I'm happy to have met you. If you have any ideas how we can help at home, just call. We want to work closely with the school.

Kroth and Edge (1997) believe that this type of conference occurs quite often. Both parent and teacher are trying to communicate and cooperate, but neither takes the time to listen to what the other has to say. In such instances, both parties leave the conference feeling that little was accomplished. Such counterproductive conferences dampen the parent's desire to return for another meeting. By the same token, the teacher does not look forward to the next meeting.

Generally speaking, it is wise to allow parents as much freedom to air their concerns as possible. After responding to these concerns, the teacher can shift the conference to matters that she wishes to discuss. Often, what the teacher wants to address in a conference corresponds to the desires of the parent, so that topics need not shift aimlessly. Should this give-and-take interchange not materialize and the parent talks for most of the session, a subsequent meeting might be scheduled, where *the teacher* has an opportunity to discuss matters she planned to raise. In such an instance, a teacher might say, "I'm pleased that we had this talk about Audrey today. Unfortunately, time will not permit me to bring up a few thoughts that I wanted to share with you. I wonder if we could set up another meeting in about two or three weeks." Such a response tells parents that the teacher is willing to listen to the parents' concerns, that she has certain time constraints, and that she has something to contribute that will serve as the structure for the next meeting.

BARRIERS TO EFFECTIVE CONFERENCES

Graduate training programs in education put little value on the development of facilitative communications skills. In teacher education, such training is of modest interest and therefore is relegated to a position of low priority. However, whether they know it or not, teachers are cast into the role of helper/facilitator—one who has a significant role to play. The acquisition of facilitative interpersonal skills, therefore, must be given higher priority in the curriculum. Teachers should read about interviewing skills and then actually *practice* them with fellow students or colleagues under expert supervision.

A block to the development of facilitative interpersonal skills may be related to the personalities and skills of supervisors and professors who educate teachers. It is not unusual for students to emulate the practices and behaviors of their mentors. Yalom (1985) observed that "pipe-smoking therapists often beget pipe-smoking patients. Patients during psychotherapy may sit, walk, talk, and even think like their therapists" (p. 17). This behavior is as true in teacher education as it is in psychotherapy.

To get a sense of how much you may have been influenced by others, write down the names of former or current supervisors, professors, or colleagues whom you emulate to some degree. Then, try to identify characteristics, behaviors, and attitudes that you have integrated into your personality or behavior. For example:

Person	Characteristics, behavior, attitudes
Ms. Swanson, teacher, supervisor	Impressed by and try to emulate the easygoing and relaxed way she related to students.
Professor Grant	Had an honest, effective, and nondefensive way of responding to questions he could not answer.

It is also informative to identify educators and supervisors who have characteristics that you hope not to emulate:

Person	Characteristics, behavior, attitudes
My 12th-grade civics teacher	Created such an intimidating class that students were afraid to ask questions.
One of my supervisors during my student teaching	He preached, moralized, and told me what to do. He had little interest in my opinion.

Teacher educators and supervisors are not always the most effective social models for their charges. Teaching, whether in college, elementary school, or elsewhere, is an *influencing* process; we are often remarkably naive about the impact our social–interpersonal conduct has on those we teach and train. In discussing the effects of social modeling in counselor education, Jakubowski-Specter, Dustin, and George (1971) observed the following:

> What a counselor educator *does* may be more influential than what he *says;* our role as a model may be more important than our role as an instructor. If a counselor educator is trying to teach genuine communication, the educator's interpersonal dealings with his students should reflect or model the kind of behavior he endorses. Through our dealings with students, we show them what we are and what we expect from people. Too often, a counselor educator verbalizes the importance of genuineness and self-disclosure while his students do not find these behaviors in their interaction with him as an advisor, practicum instructor, or professor. As models, counselor educators could more effectively facilitate learning through striving to consistently act out the behaviors they are trying to teach. This may lead to a more consistent behavior in counseling students. (pp. 248–249)

Teacher educators should be aware of the learning objectives they have formulated for their students and how their interpersonal behavior either reinforces these objectives or detracts from them. The discussion now turns to several barriers to effective interviewing *during* parent–teacher conferences.

Dealing with children for several hours a day is work, hard work, and fatigue at the end of a typical day is not uncommon. When psychologically or physically tired, it is most difficult for teachers to be attentive listeners, but inattention due to fatigue conveys a lack of interest and concern. Teachers should be aware of their tolerance levels and regulate their working day to ensure that they are alert when conferring with parents.

A factor often difficult to distinguish from physical fatigue is boredom. It is not always easy to uncover the reason for one's boredom, but one might consider the following possibilities: disinterest in listening to the problems of others, hearing essentially the same story for the sixth time, preoccupation. Different action is required depending on the causal factor(s) in operation.

Preoccupation with personal circumstance can be a barrier to effective conferencing. For example, a teacher may be going through a divorce or coping with a challenging situation that he is confronting with his own child. It is difficult to be an attentive compassionate listener when one is experiencing personal distress. Indeed, if a personal situation is so personally upsetting and distracting, one may delay parent conferences until the personal issue is less stressful.

Preoccupation may take the form of thinking ahead, that is, thinking about ones responses while the parent is talking. This is fairly common early on and generally decreases with experience and increased confidence. Transitory preoccupation is common, and is to be expected, but chronic preoccupation necessitates some serious introspection.

Strong feelings about the parent are another barrier to effective listening. Being angry with or anxious about someone with whom we are conversing cannot help but interfere with the interview. Here, again, it is helpful to be aware of the source of the anger or anxiety before taking action. Often, awareness of the source of the anger/ anxiety defuses the situation to such an extent that little else is required; the negative emotions decline in intensity and attentive listening can resume.

Professional roles can be inhibiting, although how they interfere is unclear. Some believe that distancing is necessary to allow for objectivity or perspective; others contend that professional roles, with their inevitable distancing, account for many of the ineffective interpersonal skills of people in the helping professions. Carkhuff (1968) marshaled a considerable amount of research evidence in concluding that paraprofessionals (peers with some training in human relations) perform considerably better than professionals. Paraprofessionals, he argued, are perceived as friends who understand and genuinely care, as opposed to authority figures (professionals), who are removed from a client's environment and presumably pretend to care because they receive remuneration for doing so.

Other possible barriers during conferences are differences in age, sex, race, or culture. Pacing problems and defensive behavior on the part of the interviewer can contribute to parent–teacher impasses. These variables require further attention and will be discussed in subsequent sections.

Before continuing, consider the following questions. (It is often helpful to discuss these in a group.)

1. In my experiences with others, which of the factors mentioned here have been interpersonal barriers for me? If I have overcome them, what process, technique, or person has been helpful? If I have not overcome them, perhaps someone else in the group has—but how?
2. In working with parents, which of the barriers discussed may be the most difficult for me to overcome? Which are manageable?
3. Are some of these barriers inevitable, and is there little hope that they can be changed successfully?

OTHER NEGATIVE RESPONSES FROM TEACHERS

Benjamin (1987) discusses a variety of responses considered to be nonfacilitative. *Agreement* and *disagreement* can be used to indicate that, in the teacher's opinion, the parent is right or wrong. Often, these opinions are stated before the teacher gets adequate information from the parent, or the teacher misinterprets the information.

Example: "I can't agree with you. If I were you, I'd place Robbie in a school for the deaf."

A stronger implication of good or bad is involved in *approval–disapproval* responses. The teacher is expressing a value judgment from her frame of reference. Approval can be as dangerous as disapproval; if used too much by a teacher, it can shift the focus of the conference from helping the child to achieving approval from the parents. A real tug-of-war may ensue when the parent reacts to the teacher's disapproval, like in the following example:

> *Example*: "Your suggestion of encouraging David to read more in his areas of interest is a poor one. He should be reading in a variety of different areas."

In using *ridicule or sarcasm*, the teacher condescendingly instructs the parent to demonstrate the absurdity of the parent's feelings or perceptions.

> PARENT: I'm sorry I couldn't make our last conference. You probably remember that day—it was raining so hard.
>
> TEACHER: I can understand that. You probably would have gotten wet and melted on your way over.

In *threatening* a parent, the teacher makes it clear what steps will be taken should the parent continue on the same path. In short, the parent is warned about the consequences awaiting her should she persist in her erring ways. Of all the negative responses, implicit or explicit threats are the most deplorable.

> *Example* (implicit threat): "I've told you before that it is essential that you keep me informed about David. You haven't been doing that, so we will have to see what we are going to do about it."

Defensive Behavior

Defensive behavior may be shown by either the parent or the teacher, and defensiveness by one party probably will result in some type of reciprocal defensive communication. An example of defensive communication is illustrated by the following remarks made by two teachers:

> FIRST TEACHER: I've been observing your method of trying to get kids interested and motivated in science. Your method is a

flop. The kids you work with are actually more turned off now than they were before.

SECOND TEACHER: Maybe so, but I've watched you trying to keep your kids under control. In watching you with your class, I've often wondered whether they have a teacher at all.

The first teacher's comments contributed to the second teacher's subsequent angry retort. The problem(s) they have with each other cannot be resolved as long as one or the other is made to feel inadequate and defensive. The example illustrates overt hostility and defensiveness. Sometimes the expression of angry feelings is much more subtle, for example, by using sarcasm.

It is a basic rule that whenever discernible resistance disrupts or impedes parent–teacher conferences, the exploration of such roadblocks must take precedence over other content. When a parent appears uncharacteristically quiet or annoyed, the teacher should inquire about this behavior before going on to an unrelated topic. Sensitivity and good pacing are necessary for an appropriate intervention. As an illustration, the teacher might say, "Mrs. Garvey, I noticed that in the last 15 minutes you seem reluctant to say anything. I wonder if it's because of something said earlier in our meeting . . . or perhaps it's just my imagination."

Silence is one of the most common manifestations of resistance, especially when it is preceded or followed by other avoidance cues. Superficial talk (or intellectualization) that lasts for a considerable period of time is another indication that a parent may feel resistant, as is changing the subject, ignoring the teacher's comments, arriving late for appointments, or forgetting them altogether. Filibustering, excessive questioning, and challenging the teacher about her shortcomings or flaws are other ways a parent may show defensiveness.

It is imperative that teachers understand what lies behind defensive behavior. For example, parents may be fearful of becoming involved in conferences that they feel highlight their child's shortcomings and, by association, their own inadequacies. Parents who have attended several conferences laced liberally with discussion of their child's deficiencies and problems develop a generalized dread of all conferences, whether or not their fears are justified. Misconceptions of what parent–teacher conferences are about could result in negative attitudes; parents may see them, for example, as a time to exchange social amenities or an opportunity to listen to the teachers' perceptions of the child, and not a place to express their wishes or concerns. Also, parents may fear that heavy demands will be placed on them—demands that will be overwhelming. Anger at the school, the school system, or perhaps even at the teacher, may account for resistance, as may fear that involvement with the teacher will require some sort of change in the relationship between parent and child. Finally, a parent's defensiveness during conferences may actually be a reflection of ambivalent feelings toward their child.

Defensive behavior by the parent is to be expected at times, and it is the teacher's task to deal with it effectively. Conversely, defensive behavior by the teacher can be a serious matter and is not subject to modification by parents. The teacher is the professional, and the parent is the recipient of a service. Should the teacher find himself feeling and/or acting defensively toward a parent, he would be well advised to think about the underlying reasons. Discussing the situation with an understanding friend, colleague, or supervisor can often provide fresh insights and relieve the tension a teacher feels in the parents' presence.

Interventions that are not necessarily defensive on the part of a teacher but generate defensive behavior in parents are related to *pacing* or *timing*. For example, personal inquiries concerning parents' feelings about their child are most inappropriate during the first few conferences and, in general, ought not to be asked directly. Only after meeting with the parents several times, and only when sensing that they want to discuss their innermost feelings about their child should the teacher broach the topic.

Moving too quickly can provoke anxiety; subsequent meetings will be fearful ones, if the parents show up at all. By the same token, if parents disclose their feelings of shame, guilt, or disappointment in reference to their child, the teacher should be careful not to introduce irrelevant remarks such as, "Joey was so excited last week when Santa visited the class." This type of response conveys to parents that the teacher is insensitive, feels awkward or uncomfortable because of the parents' disclosure, or, even more serious, is not interested in the parents' perceptions. As a teacher, whenever you detect that you have asked an unrelated question or given a response that bears little resemblance to what the parent has said, be sure to reflect privately on why you chose to change the subject. More often than not, a teacher is motivated to misdirect a parental response because the parents' words stimulated an anxious internal reaction. For example:

PARENT: Mrs. Goodman, I'm so glad that we are meeting today. My husband and I are having some major conflicts about Mark's tantrums at home and I am afraid that these conflicts are escalating and causing major difficulties between my husband and myself. The word "separation" came up in our last argument.

TEACHER: Actually, Mrs. Compomizzi, I'm glad you came in today, because it's such a lovely day and I want to tell you how well Mark's been doing in my class lately.

There is nothing wrong with being professional in one's work. It implies exercising good judgment and conducting oneself in a responsible and ethical manner. Unfortunately, some professional helpers equate the word "professional" with being aloof, distant, and even arrogant. This is a form of defensiveness that allows one to maintain psychological distance. Such a demeanor reflects a cold and uncaring person. Feelings of dislike, anger, or fear can lead to defensive or protective maneuvers by the teacher. Sometimes the teacher's feelings are submerged (unconscious) and not readily accessible to herself; at other times, she is aware of her feelings (e.g., anger) but not of the manifestation of related behaviors (e.g., stern look).

It is often useful to discuss issues in a small group format. If such a format is available to you, consider forming a group where you can share and receive ideas, information, and support. Before proceeding, take some time to discuss the following issues in your groups (or reflect on them individually):

- Can you think of parent–teacher situations that might make you feel or act defensively?
- Under what other circumstances in parent conferences might you feel threatened and become defensive?
- When you feel threatened, how do you tend to show it?
- When you behave defensively, how do you think others react to you?
- How do you characteristically respond to someone else who is being defensive toward you?
- Between the present group meeting and the next one, be alert to obvious and subtle examples of defensive behavior you observe in others. Also, remain aware of your own defensive feelings and behavior, and be prepared to discuss your observations at the next meeting.

Specific interviewing skills detailed in this chapter should provide a sound basis for coping with defensive behavior. Two major considerations, however, ought to be mentioned at this point:

1. Before teachers can deal with the parents' or their own defensive behavior, they must be *aware* of its existence. Awareness is the hallmark of a conscientious listener. It precedes the ability to change behavior. Teachers must be continually alert to signs of resistance in themselves and be able to recognize it when it is manifested by parents.

2. Defensive behavior should never be ignored. A teacher's defensive feelings and behavior ought to be subject to active introspection, or the teacher may wish to discuss them with a colleague or supervisor. However, as noted earlier, the teacher should sensitively probe the nature of a parent's resistance before moving on to other content. Ignoring interpersonal impasses generally leads to deeper feelings of distrust and, ultimately, to negative views of parent–teacher conferences.

LECTURING AND MORALIZING: BARRIERS TO EFFECTIVE COMMUNICATION

Lecturing or moralizing has no place in helping relationships, and it is of questionable value in other interpersonal situations as well. Some would challenge its positive value in the classroom, or perhaps even in church, when it becomes strongly moralistic or repressive.

Lecturing and moralizing share some common properties. They both imply condescension and judgment. Although teachers are generally viewed as knowledgeable and helpful professionals, those who lecture or moralize may be seen as intellectual or moral superiors, not to be questioned at best, and not caring at worst. Parents who are recipients of such behavior will act with surprise or even shock, feeling and acting defensively (revolt and arguing) or guilty and ashamed (passivity). The result is contradictory to healthy and productive interpersonal relationships.

Because lecturing and moralizing have so much in common, it is difficult to point out distinguishing characteristics. Both suggest judgment and may imply that the teacher is disapproving.

Example 1: "You know that the doctor told you that George had to have a new pair of shoes every 4 months. Not buying the shoes when he needs them can lead to permanent damage." [In this comment, the doctor is used as the authority, and guilt is generated by alluding to "permanent damage" as a consequence of the parents' negligence.]

Example 2: "We discussed working with Lucy at home during other conferences. I am disappointed that you didn't take my advice seriously. It is absolutely essential that you put aside 30 minutes each day to work with her. There are several studies that show that parents who help their children at home are able to improve children's IQ score by 10 points. I know you'll want to do what is best for your child." [This lecture includes a variety of goodies: The parent is made to feel stupid because advice given at previous sessions was not followed. The teacher registers his own sense of disapproval, thereby making the parent feel like a bad child. Authority is marshaled by citing studies indicating the parent has erred badly by acts of omission, for example, not working with the child. Finally, a parting shot from the teacher injects a dose of guilt by implying that the parent has not been acting in the best interest of her child and that she had better change.]

Communications that imply "You shouldn't have done that," "That's a stupid thing to do," "You should respect me [the teacher] more," and so on, leave the parent resentful and alienated, hardly in a mood to be accessible and cooperative.

In lecturing and moralizing, sophisticated weapons are used against the parent. Research studies, school authorities, doctors, or the teacher may be called upon to motivate or change parents' behavior. Moralizing can be made even more potent, and is thereby distinguishable from lecturing, by using religious tenets. Teachers with strong religious convictions must be careful not to use personal beliefs to manipulate parents, as illustrated in the following somewhat extreme example:

"We know that in God's eyes, some people are born inferior and because of that, I can see why you find it hard to accept Sam the way he is."

On rare occasions, personal religious beliefs are used by teachers in grossly misguided efforts to be helpful. Infrequently, a small minority of those in the helping professions are so caught up by their missionary zeal, combined with a genuine desire to be helpful, that they try to proselytize for their particular sect. For example:

> "I know how anxious and depressed you are about your child's disability and your home situation that keeps getting worse. It seems like there is little hope—a very bleak future ahead. By the way, a religious organization that I belong to has been of help to others who are in despair. Our next meeting is Thursday. Why don't you come along with me and see what you think?"

Although these remarks cannot be classified as moralizing in the strict sense, because they do not imply a judgment, personal religious beliefs—as well as personal beliefs about such issues as abortion or women's rights—have no place in parent–teacher conferences. There is a significant difference between trying to coax a personal friend to a meeting of a religious group and the parent of a child with special needs. When referrals are required, teachers should make them to other *professional* services and agencies, not to religious or quasi-religious sects, faith healers, and the like.

Moralizing or lecturing represents the antithesis of effective interpersonal communications, as illustrated by the following poignant remarks by Benjamin (1974):

> The interviewee is trapped. To surrender is to admit defeat. To resist is to declare himself an outlaw. Shall he bend the knee or raise his head in challenge? Thus beleaguered, he may act in a number of ways, but the chances are it will be acting, pretense. What is really happening within himself he is sure to keep well hidden. The foe is too formidable, the pressure too great, for anything but playacting or evasion. True, it may not always be playacting; the "culprit" may genuinely feel guilty and be shocked by his own behavior. Moralizing has been known to work. (p. 139)

SILENCES

In contrast to Eastern cultures, Western cultures find silence between people barely tolerable. Because silence is viewed as an empty situation without meaning, when it does occur between two people or in a small group, those involved often feel uncomfortable. However, people engaged in helping others must appreciate and be able to use and tolerate silences. Before continuing, take 20–30 minutes to discuss the following related issues in your group:

1. How you *feel* when there are periods of silence between you and another person.
2. How you *feel* when there are periods of silence in a small group.
3. What would your *feelings* be if the discussion at this moment fell silent? (Should silences occur while doing this exercise, reflect upon and then discuss your interpretation of them.)
4. Consider situations in which you have been keenly aware of silences and how you (internally) responded to them (e.g., in a doctor's waiting room, in the teacher's lunchroom, on elevators, sitting next to a stranger on a plane).

For people who conduct interviews, silences should be considered a positive form of communication. Beginning interviewers feel they must talk when pauses or silences occur, and an uneasy sense of wasting time or not doing a good job causes them to make inappropriate comments or ask unnecessary questions. Unfortunately, there are no rules about how long is too long for a period of silence. Each situation has to be assessed on its own merit. Silence is worthwhile only as long as it is communicating something or serving some function. It can best be understood if the meaning of the pause and the context in which it occurs are clear. A high degree of sensitivity is required for the teacher to know when to remain quiet and when to make an appropriate remark. Benjamin (1987) illustrates the many meanings silences can have:

> Silence may express the desire to listen rather than speak. Silence may mean evasion and escape. Silence may indicate resistance, hostility, aggression. Silence may, signify lack of interest and even boredom. Silence often expresses confusion, lack of direction, lost bearings. Silence may, of course, communicate ineffable grief that should command our respect. It may ultimately denote deep concentration and thought . . . that we ought not interrupt. In short, silence conveys many varied messages that we must lean to decipher and respond to in accordance with the interpretation we have reached. (p. 42)

Sensitivity is generally acquired as one gains experience with the "sounds of silence," but a review of silent behavior and what it may mean can increase awareness, which in turn can increase the teacher's comfort with it.

Strong emotions may emerge, temporarily interrupting the flow of a parent's verbalization. Such emotions may be the result of the discussion of painful events, the recall of emotionally laden situations, or sudden insights. According to Schulman (1978), silence during the early part of an interview may reflect a parent's embarrassment, resistance, or fear of what the teacher is thinking. Generally, as the interview progresses, silences gradually take on a more supportive meaning and serve as a medium for emotional expression and thought. It is essential for teachers to relay to parents that they can be quiet and still be liked, accepted, and respected. They may use periods of silence to delve deeply into their feelings, to struggle with alternative courses of action, or to weigh a decision.

Silence can be a consequence of an apparent search for words or an attempt to clarify thoughts and feelings. For a teacher to interrupt during a thoughtful silent period can interfere with the parents' struggle to organize their thoughts. It is not unreasonable to expect parental silence after they have been given some unanticipated or negative news about their child. This pause allows the parents to contemplate what has just been said. As noted earlier, when a teacher senses that long silences with a particular parent are an expression of resistance or defensiveness, it is the teacher's responsibility to deal actively with the situation. If she believes that she understands the nature of the resistance, a response such as the following may be appropriate:

> "I wonder if the long silences we have been having lately are because I suggested at our last meeting that you might want to consult a psychologist. If so, I would very much like to know your thoughts about our last meeting."

Should the teacher be quite sure of the resistance but not know its source, the teacher might say,

> "I'm sure that we are both aware of the times we sit here not saying anything to each other. I sense a feeling of tension between us but I don't know what is causing it. Do you have any idea?"

Except as a manifestation of defensive behavior, teachers should view silences in a much more positive fashion than is generally the case in our culture. Silences, more often than not, give parents a chance to rest or to reflect and organize their thoughts. Also, since teachers' primary professional activity is to teach—in which speaking is essential—they may not be inclined to value silences or to find them easy to tolerate. Thus, they should consider the virtues of silence and its appropriate use.

OVERTALK

Teachers are trained to convey information, to communicate ideas, to answer questions, and to ask them. To engage in such activities, teachers must be verbal; therefore, they talk more, and appropriately so, than the children they teach, although good teachers also listen.

When teachers confer with parents, the pendulum should swing in the direction of increased listening, and talking becomes a secondary activity. This shift may be a problem for some teachers, as it appears that students who select teaching as a profession enjoy talking, teaching, and instructing. In my experience, students in teacher training programs appear to be fairly verbal. If teachers are more accustomed to talking than listening, they must make a concerted effort during parent–teacher conferences to control their speech and concentrate on what is being said. Hetznecker et al. (1978) believe that overtalk can best be unlearned in simulated conferences where role playing is emphasized. This change is critical, the authors feel, because both parent and teacher in their respective roles vis-à-vis the child are accustomed to talk more than to listen. "Advice, correction, admonishment, persuasion, information giving, and questioning are the adult techniques both parent and teacher direct at children. When relating to parents, a teacher needs to shift to a more receptive, attentive mode which emphasizes listening" (p. 366).

In defense of excessively verbal teachers, I should mention that professional helpers in other fields also talk more than they listen, particularly during their initial stage of training. Overtalk tends to decrease with training, in which feedback from supervisors and peers highlights both positive and negative aspects of an interviewing style.

Overtalk may be symptomatic of a teacher's nervousness or represent a characteristic most of us share, namely, the tendency to give advice prematurely. Unlike counselors and psychotherapists, teachers do not have opportunities to work on their interviewing style in their training programs because of the secondary importance given to helpful interpersonal communication in teacher training programs.

A way to ascertain one's talking-to-listening ratio is to record role-played interviews. To add a realistic dimension to the self-evaluation, record a few actual parent–teacher conferences, being sure to obtain the parents' permission first. Tell the parent's why you intend to record the session and how the recording will be used (e.g., for your review after the conference to help you improve your conferencing skills).

Another method commonly used to train social workers requires the interviewer to write down as accurately as possible what each person in the interview said. This is called a process recording, of which the following is a brief illustration:

MRS. BROWN: I feel awful about Terry's performance in school. He is falling farther and farther behind.

TEACHER: I can sense your concern about Terry's lack of progress. What makes the situation even worse is your feeling that your son is losing ground that he won't be able to make up.

MRS. BROWN (*moving uncomfortably in her chair*): Yes, and the more he gets behind, the more his father and I push him, to work harder. But the more we push him the less he seems to do. I'm just at my wits' end with Terry—what do you think I ought to do?

TEACHER (*feeling uncomfortable, that she must come up with a solution*): Well, maybe what you can do is to tell him about his other friends who are doing well in school because they work hard on their subjects. You could also tell him about some famous people who were very poor but overcame their problems by hard work and concentration. Another possibility would be to have him evaluated by our psychological consultant. There may be a psychological reason for his lack of progress.

MRS. BROWN (*looking confused*): Well, we told him so many times about his friends, Jerry and Roger, and how well they do in school because of their hard work. I think it's a good idea to talk to Terry about some people who have made it and the hard work it took to get there but—do you think there is something psychologically wrong with our son?

And so on, and so on.

As you listen to a tape recording, go over a process recording, or if you are simply reflecting on an earlier meeting, keep the following points in mind:

1. Did you find yourself giving advice inappropriately? That is, did you offer advice before you really understood what the parents were saying?
2. In your eagerness to respond, did you catch yourself interrupting the parents?
3. Do you detect indications that you repeated yourself unnecessarily?
4. Were there indications that you tended to overelaborate a point? If so, try to recall your feelings during the conference.
5. Did you find yourself repeating statements during uncomfortable silences?
6. Did you catch yourself interrupting a parent because you were afraid of forgetting the point you wanted to make?
7. Did you have a tendency to overelaborate when you were fearful of the parent, thereby giving him less time to talk and thus reducing your anxiety?

TEACHERS' SELF-DISCLOSURE

Expected responses of parents during conferences are the expression of their reactions to the teacher's observations about the child's progress, their perceptions of how the child relates to other family members at home, their own feelings and those of other family members toward the child, and so on. These verbalizations characterize a level of self-disclosure (or personal sharing) that is critical to cooperative and helpful parent–teacher conferences. This is the parents' contribution to the conference.

Although some degree of self-disclosure by the parent is important, the same cannot be said of the teacher. This issue is somewhat more complex in that a teacher's more circumspect comments about his social and professional life and his reactions to a parent or a child are appropriate and often turn out to be helpful. In contrast, self-disclosures that dwell at great length on a teacher's educational achievement, professional reputation, marital problems, or problems with his children, confuse and bewilder parents. Under these circumstances, the parent is placed in the position of counselor. Although there is merit to limited personal sharing in parent–teacher conferences, a teacher's indiscriminate self-disclosure serves the needs of the wrong person.

The following exercise allows you to examine a teacher's self-disclosing responses. Although I have given my views, I invite your perception of which responses are appropriate and which are not. Also, in your groups, give examples and discuss what you consider to be proper and improper self-disclosing comments during a parent–teacher conference.

1a. *Inappropriate*: "You know, I can relate to what you just said. Sometimes my boyfriend treats me as if I don't exist. It really bugs me, but I'm afraid if I mention this to him, he might leave me."

1b. *Appropriate*: "Yes, I know what you mean. There was a time when I had to juggle a job, a growing family, and school at the same time. It must make you feel like you're pretty much under the gun." [This response returns the focus on the parent.]

2a. *Inappropriate*: "Boy, I am really angry! Ms. Kern, who just left, called me an incompetent teacher when I try to spend extra time with her boy. Sometimes I just don't feel appreciated in this job." [Not only is the self-disclosure in poor taste, but also the teacher's remarks raise an ethical issue; what is it?]

2b. *Appropriate*: "The pleasure you feel when you help David reminds me of how good I feel when I take the time to work with my son."

3a. *Inappropriate*: "I know what you mean. Dealing with in-laws can be a real pain. My mother-in-law really makes me feel inadequate. If I let her, she would mother my kids and husband to death. She often makes me feel left out."

3b. *Appropriate* [in response to a question]: "Yes, the teaching profession can be demanding. The pressures pay off, though, when you see kids improving and liking what they are doing."

TERMINATION

Ending a conference is generally not difficult, although it can be a problem in some circumstances. A parent's behavior may reflect an anxious need to keep talking, or perhaps a need to have someone with whom to talk, to compensate for loneliness. At other times, it may indicate a more generalized difficulty with termination, a holdover perhaps from an earlier experience, when it was traumatic to end an important relationship. Also, parents may be reluctant to end a conference because opportunities to talk with their child's teacher are rare, and they want to get in all the time they can. If this is the case, the teacher may wish to consider scheduling more frequent meetings. However, the teacher must still end the conference.

Parent–teacher conferences are often circumscribed by time. These time limits are usually the result of realistic constraints, such as a teacher's other duties, a policy determined by the school, or a teacher's thoughts on the adequate amount of time for a conference.

Whenever possible, rigid time constraints under all conditions should be avoided. Semiannual or quarterly conferences designed to communicate a student's progress may be scheduled for a 20-minute time period. Conferences designed to discuss issues in more depth should run longer (perhaps 30–40 minutes).

For some interviewers, beginners in particular, closing is not easy. The teacher may be fearful of giving the impression of pushing the parent out—and depending on how termination is handled, a parent may indeed have this feeling.

Benjamin (1987) believes that the closing phase of an interview is critical, and two basic factors should be kept in mind: (1) Both people in the interview should be aware that closing is taking place and accept it, the interviewer in particular; (2) during termination, no new material should be discussed, because this phase should focus on what has already taken place. If fresh information or concerns emerge during closing, another interview will have to be scheduled.

There are important reasons for deferring new material during the final minutes of a conference. The teacher may have to keep another appointment and will therefore find it difficult to be attentive if the conference continues. He may also become covertly angry at the parent for coming up with new material that could have been introduced earlier. New information may be introduced (in fact, there is no way to avoid its introduction), but it can be deferred to the next meeting: "What you just mentioned is certainly important for us to discuss. Unfortunately, our time has run out, but let's plan to discuss it first thing at our next conference."

Parents may not necessarily know how much time is at their disposal during a conference. In this instance, the teacher can help by indicating that time will be up shortly: "Well our time is just about up. Is there anything else you'd care to mention before we close, so that we can put it on our agenda for next time?" A teacher may wish to restate the gist of the discussion and, if necessary, comment about the focus of the next meeting:

"I'm glad we had a chance to go over Ray's academic work. We both seem to agree that his language development and reading are coming along. We also talked about his problems in math, a concern that we plan to watch. At our next meeting, let's spend

some time on how our plans to help Ray seem to affect his attitude
and his ability to complete his math assignments. Does this make
sense to you?" [It is always helpful to ask for the parents' collaboration.]

The termination of a conference should not be taken lightly. What
occurs during the closing stage is likely to determine the parents' experience of the interview as a whole. Teachers should leave enough time
for closing so that they do not find themselves rushed, since this might
create the impression that the parent is being evicted. In general, the
task of ending an interview becomes easier as the teacher appreciates
its importance and learns to feel comfortable with it.

This chapter has explored several basic principles of conferencing.
Chapter 6 includes additional core aspects of the interview and adds
specific strategies that teachers should find helpful in conducting parent conferences.

6

Useful Strategies in Working with Parents of Children with Disabilities

Chapter 5 examined some of the conceptual principles involved in conducting effective parent–teacher conferences. This chapter explores a variety of strategies generally used in interviewing/conferencing. Where appropriate, role-playing exercises are included that allow the reader to practice the skills discussed.

ESTABLISHING RAPPORT

The word "rapport" is thrown around more often by professionals, educators, and students in the helping professions than a basketball at a neighborhood pickup game. It is a central concept in the context of interpersonal relationships. To put it succinctly, rapport in the interviewing process refers to a comfortable yet rewarding (productive) meeting

157

between two or more people. It is enhanced by good listening and responding, as well as the experience of acceptance that results in mutual feelings of trust and respect. Intuitively, both parent and teacher generally sense when rapport between them is good and when it is not. This intuitive feeling exists in other interpersonal encounters as well, for example, between a teacher and his supervisor, and between colleagues, students, and social friends. It is important to accept the notion that it is the teacher's responsibility to establish good rapport, not the parent's (Heaton, 1998). We tend to avoid acquaintances when we sense a lack of mutual caring and respect. Heaton firmly believes that strained relationships become bad because of the absence of rapport, whereas good ones are characterized by rapport.

As discussed in Chapter 5, it is essential to confront the issue of rapport (if it is lacking) before proceeding to other concerns; that is, if the teacher experiences a parent as tense, noncommunicative, or withdrawn, it is important to address this discomfort before proceeding. If, for example, the teacher observes that Mr. and Mrs. Higgins are less talkative than usual, he can say something like: "I notice that you are less involved in our meeting today than you have been during previous conferences. I wonder if something happened in our last meeting that you may have questions about . . . or perhaps I am completely off base with my observation, but it does seem as if you are preoccupied today." In attempting to understand what might account for a suspected impasse, you might consider the following causative factors (some of these factors have been mentioned previously):

1. You have a strong dislike for the parents' child, who happens to be the most demanding and exasperating youngster you have had in class in years. Your sense of frustration with the child makes it difficult to be comfortable with the parents.
2. You sense that there is an adverse reaction to you, but you are not sure why. (Be careful about personalizing parental behavior—parents may be grumpy about a flat tire they had earlier.)
3. You know that the parents view their child's educational program with considerable skepticism.
4. Either you or the parents are preoccupied with events not related to the conference (see item 2).
5. You sense that the parents are uncomfortable talking about their child, perhaps because they worry about bad news.

6. You are threatened by the parents because you perceive that their professional status equals or exceeds yours.

7. You are threatened by the parents because you know they are sophisticated about their child's exceptionality.

Sometimes, just understanding why rapport is poor between the teacher and the parents is sufficient. For example, knowing that the parents are preoccupied with a personal crisis, the teacher may wish to acknowledge her understanding that the parents are experiencing a problem, give them an opportunity to discuss it, if they wish, or re-schedule another appointment at some future date. Understanding that parents are displeased with their child's educational program may be unsettling and pose a personal threat to the teacher. However, per-haps this dissatisfaction reflects the parents' excessive concern about the education of their children and their tendency to be critical of most things.

This awareness not only allows the teacher to feel less threatened but also provides cues about how she might work with the parents. For example, the teacher might keep excessively concerned or overly critical parents well informed of the educational program developed for their child (which is usually the case during the IEP conference). If appropriate, she may even solicit their input, knowing that they will be less critical of a program they helped develop. Parents' behavior is of-ten a manifestation of anxiety. By intelligently and cooperatively working with parents, the teacher can reduce their anxiety to the ex-tent that at least a minimal level of rapport is possible.

When the teacher senses that anxiety arises when he begins to talk about the parents' child, he might consider saying something like, "I'm not sure that I'm right, but it seems that whenever we begin to talk about Judy, you seem to tense up," or "You seem to get an overly con-cerned look on your face whenever we begin to discuss Judy. Am I right or am I off the track?" However, if the teacher makes such a com-ment, he should have enough time to listen to the parents' response.

Such an inquiry can open the door to a frank discussion of the par-ents' feelings and perceptions about their child. It may be a relief for them to discuss secretly held concerns with an empathic listener. Should their concerns roughly correspond to those generally faced by parents of children with disabilities, the teacher can, at least for a few meetings, help them to verbalize their worries. In this way, the parent–teacher relationship can proceed with a feeling of enhanced rapport. However, if the problems are beyond the scope of the teacher's comfort or expertise, he should listen attentively and then suggest that the parents consider talking with someone who is more qualified. Indications of psychological problems that require the attention of a mental health professional include the following:

1. When a parent feels compelled to abuse her child psychologically or physically (there are reporting requirements relative to abusive situations).
2. When a parent implies that the child's existence is the cause of considerable family discord.
3. When a parent is unable to shake the feeling that the child is another indication of her inadequacy as a person.
4. When a parent's guilt over bearing a child with a disability is unbearable to the extent that she has considered suicide.
5. When a parent reports that since the birth of the child, nightmares have become commonplace.
6. When parents comment that the child is difficult and an embarrassment, and they find it difficult to be in her presence.

Whenever the teacher is unsure of the magnitude of the parents' reaction, she should consider discussing her observations with the school psychologist or some other available psychological consultant.

It is difficult to be prescriptive when we consider human interactions. Some teachers would be comfortable if their responses to parents could be learned in a programmed fashion. In establishing rapport or confronting the lack of it, there simply is no substitute for a perceptive, sensitive teacher with good judgment. There are rare instances when confronting a situation will damage rapport even more; other times, it will help, but making believe that rapport exists when it is problematic, or hoping that it will improve by itself, is simply unproductive. A sensitive probe will lay the foundation for a more gratifying relationship between teacher and parent.

RAPPORT AND CULTURAL DIVERSITY

Our multicultural society makes it imperative that teachers understand how cultural differences between parents and teachers can affect conferences. For example, teachers should be aware that some minority parents may be anxious or suspicious during initial meetings, especially if their experiences with such face-to-face meetings have been limited. Simpson (1996) provides an illustration of how a teacher's lack of experience and cultural expectations can lead to unwanted behaviors: "One Hispanic father who had been asked to attend a progress report conference about his son confided that he had punished his child prior to the meeting because he assumed that it (the meeting) was called in response to the boys bad classroom behavior" (p. 76).

Small talk at the beginning of a conference may be viewed suspiciously by some minority group members, because such behavior may be indicative of a delaying tactic or the teacher's wishes to avoid an unpleasant topic. In contrast, other parents may want to discuss more socially oriented topics for a few minutes before addressing school-related concerns (Simpson, 1996).

Sometimes, language can impede rapport, either in instances when the parent and teacher speak different languages or when parents have limited language ability. The presence of a translator or interpreter may help communication, but it can also hinder it. According to Barnwell and Day (1996), an interpreter should be trained in early childhood education, cross-cultural interpretation, and be fluent in both languages. One should be cautious of using family members as interpreters, especially if sensitive and confidential issues are discussed. Randall-David (1989, cited in Barnwell & Day, 1996) provides a more in-depth discussion of how one might constructively use interpreters during conferences.

Teachers should avoid complex sentences, slang, professional jargon, or technical language when conferring with parents from different cultures who may not be fluent in English. Furthermore, teachers should be wary of talking down to them. The rate of a teacher's speech should be adjusted so that parents can understand what is being said. Repeating sentences when parents seem puzzled is a good idea, but it should be done in a pleasant (not irritable tone), so that parents are not reluctant to ask further questions. Barnwell and Day (1996) suggest that professionals (1) have some familiarity with special terminology in other languages, (2) have a positive tone, (3) avoid being patronizing or judgmental, (4) repeat critical information, (5) provide a rationale for suggestions, and (6) provide family members with material written in their language, if possible.

Gender can also be an issue in working with culturally diverse populations. In this regard, Simpson (1996) notes that some Hispanics may be reluctant to be advised by a woman. Also, based solely on the issue of gender, members of certain minority groups may avoid eye contact.

There are a variety of resources that will help teachers become more aware of the unique aspects of various cultures such as the chapter "Cultural Reactions to Childhood Disability and Subcultural Variation" in Seligman and Darling (1997); Shea and Bauer's (1991) book, *Parents and Teachers of Children with Exceptionalities;* the classic, now in its second edition, *Ethnicity and Family Therapy* (McGoldrick et al., 1996); or Harry's (1992) *Cultural Diversity, Families, and the Special Education System.*

In conferencing with parents, teachers may be well advised to follow the suggestions by Lynch (1992), so that their interactions with culturally diverse persons are successful:

1. Self-awareness: The professional should first be able to articulate the relevant norms, values, and beliefs of his or her *own* culture.
2. Awareness of other cultures in general.
3. Awareness of other cultures' views of children and child rearing, disability, family roles and structures, healing practices, and intervention by professionals.
4. Cross-cultural communications, including verbal and nonverbal messages such as eye contact, proximity and touching, gestures, and listening skills.
5. Acknowledgment of cultural differences.

In attempting to cope with parents who miss scheduled conferences or seem reluctant to schedule them, keep in mind Harry's (1992) admonition that professionals must recognize that issues of survival for some families are given precedence over other concerns, such as education. Parents with needs for food, clothing, shelter, health care, and safety will not have the time or energy, or interest, to discuss educational issues, even if they have deep affection for their child. Other cautions include not discrediting folk theories or remedies unless you *know* they are harmful, asking direct questions only if appropriate to the parents' cultural and linguistic expectations, including extended family members or others in a conference if they are normally part of the support system of the family, and being willing to tolerate silences (Kavanagh & Kennedy, 1992).

Above all, try to keep an open mind and regard minority group parents as potentially diverse as the majority Caucasian society in the United States. Stereotypical beliefs attributed to all members of a cultural minority reflect a prejudiced way of thinking that can impede collaborative parent–teacher relations.

NONVERBAL BEHAVIOR
AND PARALINGUISTICS

Most authors who have written on counseling, interpersonal behavior, or interviewing eventually address the issue of nonverbal behavior. In relating to another person, we depend heavily, perhaps at a somewhat less than conscious level, on nonverbal or paralinguistic cues to interpret verbal messages. An early study designed to judge whether one person likes another revealed that a person's actual words contribute only 7% to the impression of being liked or disliked, whereas voice cues account for 38%, and facial cues, 55% (Mehrabian, 1971). This research revealed that when facial cues are incompatible with spoken words, facial expressions are believed more than words. According to Knapp (1978), nonverbal gestures can confirm, deny, or confuse a verbal message. For example, if a parent admits to being comfortable during a conference, yet develops a growing rash on her face and throat, one can surmise that she is anxious. The rash fading or disappearing is a clue that the nervousness is subsiding.

For purposes of definition, "nonverbal behavior" includes general body movements, gestures, and facial expressions; "paralinguistic behavior" is manifested in tone of voice, inflection, spacing of words, emphasis, and pauses. Another dimension of nonverbal behavior is body language, which includes the distance between people and the orientation or direction of the body (proxemics) as well as its motion (kinesics) (Heaton, 1998). Schulman (1974) has developed a scale (see Figure 6.1) that can be used to tabulate the nonverbal behavior of people who are being observed. The scale also incorporates units on eye contact and attending behavior.

The idea that words are often intended to obscure a true feeling or a particular meaning has gone beyond hypothesis; that is, nonverbal cues do, in fact, more accurately reflect a person's inner life than what one says. Since this belief has been substantiated by a considerable amount of research (Knapp, 1978; Egan, 1998; Benjamin, 1987; Ivey, 1983), it is reasonable for those in the helping professions (including education) to become knowledgeable about and alert to nonverbal behavior.

For most of us, the discrepancy between verbal and nonverbal behavior (e.g., someone says he feels perfectly comfortable in your presence, but he sits rigidly in a chair with his arms and legs crossed) is not traumatic, although it is perhaps confusing and at times annoying. There is, however, some evidence that such double communication can have a devastating effect on children, who see their parents as

FIGURE 6.1. Measurement scale: Listening and responding skills. From Schulman (1974). Copyright 1974. All rights reserved. Reprinted by permission of Allyn & Bacon.

Directions: Place a check (√) next to the rating that most closely approximates your observation of the interviewer's behavior.

Eye contact: Maintains appropriate gaze, which is not a stare, but does not look away.
1. Gaze is persistent and comfortable. ____
2. Gaze is appropriate most of the time. ____
3. Shifts gaze a little too often. ____
4. Frequently shifts gaze. ____
5. Persistently shifts gaze or stares. ____

Attending: Maintains appropriate posture; bends slightly forward from waist; maintains comfortable distance from client.
1. Persistently shifts position and moves about. ____
2. Frequently shifts position and moves about. ____
3. Shifts position a little too often. ____
4. Most of the time maintains appropriate posture. ____
5. Persistently maintains appropriate posture. ____

Hand gestures: Moves hands slowly and appropriately; gestures appear to be comfortable.
1. Gestures are persistently comfortable and appropriate. ____
2. Gestures are usually comfortable and appropriate. ____
3. Some signs of "jerky" hand movements, which are disturbing. ____
4. Tense, sudden movements frequently occur. ____
5. Persistently uses inappropriate and annoying hand gestures. ____

Facial expression: Smiles or shows other expressions that are appropriate and pleasant.
1. Persistently maintains unpleasant and inappropriate facial expressions. ____
2. Usually maintains unpleasant and inappropriate facial expression. ____
3. Occasionally has unpleasant and inappropriate facial expression. ____
4. Usually maintains pleasant and appropriate facial expression. ____
5. Persistently maintains pleasant and appropriate facial expression. ____

Voice tone: Voice is pleasant, sounds relaxed, and has appropriate volume for hearing.
1. Persistently has unpleasant tone that varies in loudness, either too loud or too low. ____
2. Usually has unpleasant tone that varies in loudness. ____
3. Occasionally has pleasant tone with appropriate volume. ____
4. Usually has pleasant tone with appropriate volume. ____
5. Persistently has pleasant tone with appropriate volume. ____

Comment: Write a brief comment about the interviewer that you think the supervisor should know.

communicating two contradictory messages (e.g., a mother telling her child she loves him while physically moving away).

An enormously useful skill for teachers, then, would be the ability to read nonverbal cues. These cues either augment what teachers are hearing or provide insight into a feeling or attitude that may be hidden. Effective listening includes the effort to hear what is not being verbalized, what may be hinted at, what is being held back, and what lies beneath the surface (Benjamin, 1987). As noted in Chapter 5, we hear with our ears, but we listen with our mind, eyes, heart, skin, and guts (Ekman, 1964).

Teachers need to be cautious in their interpretation of nonverbal cues. The same behavior manifested by two different people may have vastly different meanings. Interviewers often make a "perception check" on what they think they are perceiving. For example, a teacher may comment to a parent: "I hear you saying that you are pleased with George's progress but your facial expression leads me to believe that you are not entirely satisfied. Am I reading you right or am I off base?" This type of check enables the parent to confirm or refute the teacher's observation.

As teachers gain experience and become more aware of nonverbal behaviors, their ability to interpret and respond effectively to these cues will grow. However, teachers should be aware of traps such as the one in which a misguided psychologist ascribed (in a Sunday supplement) specific meanings to specific nonverbal behaviors. This person undoubtedly wrote the article for its entertainment value and actually included a series of rather innocuous and amusing behaviors. Nevertheless, pronouncements in which the behavior and interpretation appear to be inseparable should be regarded cautiously. Especially now, with our improved understanding of culture and behavior, interpretations of nonverbal behavior must include knowledge of cultural factors.

Egan (1986, 1998) extends the concept of verbal listening to include nonverbal behavior. He developed three exercises to help sharpen the reader's perceptual and communication skills.

Exercise 1: Body Language

You are in a meeting, observing your fellow group members. You observe, at one time or another, the following nonverbal or paralinguistic (voice-related) behaviors. Without any further context, try to indicate what possible meanings each of these behaviors may have. Try to find more than one meaning for each behavior.

1. A person nods his head up and down.
2. A person turns her head rapidly in a certain direction.
3. A person smiles slightly.
4. A person's lower lip is quivering.
5. A person speaks in a high-pitched voice.

   6. A person's voice is monotonous.
   7. A person suddenly opens his eyes wide.
   8. A person keeps her eyes lowered as she speaks to someone else.
   9. A person's nostrils are flaring.
  10. A person raises one eyebrow.
  11. A person shrugs his shoulders.
  12. A person has her shoulders forced back.
  13. A person has his arms folded tightly across his chest.
  14. A person is waving her arms.
  15. A person is holding his chair tightly with his hands.
  16. A person hides part of her body with her hands.
  17. A person's breathing is quite irregular.
  18. A person inhales quickly.
  19. A person digs his heels into the floor.
  20. A person continuously moves her legs back and forth.
  21. A person sits with her arms and legs folded tightly.
  22. A person is constantly squirming.
  23. A person holds her body bent to one side.
  24. A person has a tic.
  25. A person is getting pale. (Egan, 1986, pp. 100–101)

Compare your meanings with those of a partner, or share them with all members of the group. How many different meanings are associated with each kind of behavior? What are the implications of this fact?

Notice that most of these behaviors have more than one possible interpretation. For this reason, both verbal and nonverbal behavior must be interpreted in light of the total communication: the verbal and nonverbal behavior of the speaker and the context in which his communication is taking place.

Exercise 2: The Importance of Nonverbal Cues for Verbal Communication

The purpose of this exercise is to provide some idea of how much one depends on nonverbal cues in the interpretation of verbal messages.

Choose a partner from among your fellow group members. Sit facing your partner. *Close your eyes.* Have a 2- or 3-minute conversation on some topic you agree to discuss; remember to keep your eyes closed during the entire conversation.

Afterward, share the feelings that emerged during the conversation. What nonverbal cues did you miss the most? In what ways was the conversation stilted and awkward?

Exercise 3: Listening to Nonverbal and Paralinguistic Cues

The purpose of this exercise is to become more sensitive to nonverbal and paralinguistic cues and messages that may confirm, punctuate, emphasize, modulate, or otherwise modify the verbal messages of the speaker and thus contain the real message. For instance, if the speaker raises his voice (paralinguistic cue) and pounds on the table (nonverbal behavior) while delivering an angry message, then both cues underscore and emphasize his anger. However, if the speaker says very hesitantly (paralinguistic cue), while fidgeting with his hands (nonverbal cue), that yes, he would like to go out to dinner that night, these cues contain the real message that contradicts the verbal one.

The following list provides a fairly comprehensive sample of important nonverbal behaviors of which an interviewer should be aware:

- *bodily behavior*, such as posture, body movements, and gestures.
- *facial expression*, such as smiles, frowns, raised eyebrows, and twisted lips.
- *voice-related behavior*, such as tone of voice, pitch, voice level, intensity, inflection, spacing of words, emphases, pauses, silences, and fluency.
- *observable autonomic physiological responses*, such as quickened breathing, the development of a temporary rash, blushing, paleness, and pupil dilation.
- *physical characteristics*, such as fitness, height, weight, and complexion.
- *general appearance*, such as grooming and dress. (Egan, 1998, p. 70)

Divide into groups of four (members *a*, *b*, *c*, and *d*). Members *a* and *b* should spend 5 or 6 minutes discussing what they like and do not like about their present interpersonal style (or any other topic relevant to the training). Members *c* and *d* act as observers. While *a* and *b* are speaking, *c* and *d* should take written notes on *a* and *b*'s nonverbal and paralinguistic behavior, being careful not to over-interpret it. After 5 or 6 minutes, *c* and *d* should report to *a* and *b* the highlights of the observed behavior. Then roles are switched, and the process is repeated. Some examples of typical feedback are as follows:

"Most of the time you spoke very quickly, in spurts. It gave me a feeling of tension or nervousness."

"You sat very still throughout the dialogue. Your hands remained folded in your lap the whole time, and there was almost no bodily movement. The position made you look very proper, and it gave me an impression of shyness or rigidity."

"When you talked about being a very sensitive person, one who is easily hurt, you began to stumble over your words a bit. The message seemed to be that you are sensitive about being so sensitive."

"You tapped your left foot almost constantly."

"You put your hand to your mouth a great deal. It gave me the impression of hesitance on your part."

"When *b* began to talk hesitantly about being shy, you leaned back and even moved your chair back a bit. I'm not sure whether you were showing him that he made you uncomfortable, or whether you were easing *off*, giving him room to speak."

"You broke eye contact a great deal when you were talking about yourself, but not when you were listening."

"You were so relaxed—at times, you even slouched a bit—that you almost gave me the impression that you were uninterested in the whole task."

"You seemed so relaxed, open, and attentive to what Karen was saying. It made it easier to talk about more personal issues."

Compelling, recent research suggests that facial expressions can be precisely determined, so that it is virtually impossible for someone to fake an emotion. A new computer program is so precise that it can decipher facial muscles that are either an accurate reflection of an emotion or an attempt to deceive or keep an emotion hidden (*Pittsburgh Post-Gazette*, 1998). Therefore, during a facial analysis, it would be difficult to feign depression or anxiety; conversely, it would be difficult to hide it. This new procedure highlights our sometimes intuitive feeling that someone's denial of anxiety is confusing, because we are picking up anxiety in that person's facial expression.

MINIMAL ENCOURAGES TO TALK

The interview may be thought of as a give-and-take meeting between two people, where one person is generally (but not always) a professional helper of some kind and the other is in need of information or assistance. Before this mutual exchange, it is generally the responsibility of the interviewer (the teacher) to encourage the interviewee (the parent) to talk, to express as fully as possible the reasons for the visit, or to express any concerns that arise during the conference. It is also most helpful to encourage parents to respond to the teacher's assessment, evaluation, or impressions (e.g., I'd welcome any reactions you have to what I said.").

A teacher may impede the parent's full expression by saying too much or by intervening inappropriately (poor timing). Particularly during initial meetings, or during the first few minutes of a particular meeting, it is the teacher's task to stay out of the parent's way and, at the same time, convey her attentiveness.

By providing limited structure, minimal encouragement to talk will reinforce the parent's opportunity to communicate as well as convey the fact that the teacher is listening. Examples of minimal encouragement include the following:

"Could you tell me more?"
"Where would you like to begin today?"
"Oh?" "So?" "Then?"
"And?"
"Mm-hm." "Uh-huh."
The repetition of one or two key words.
Simple restatement of the parent's last comment ("You are worried about your husband's reaction to your son's misbehavior").
Silence (accompanied by nonverbal indicators of attentiveness, e.g., making eye contact, leaning forward)

For example, consider Benjamin's (1987) analysis of the utterance, "Mm-hm." By using "Mm-hm" the interviewer is saying, "Go on, I'm with you; I'm listening and following you," as well as indicating approval of what the parent is saying.

Of course, we can communicate in a positive or negative vein by using paralinguistic (how words are expressed) or nonverbal behavior (e.g., raising an eyebrow). As a general rule, minimal encouragement (or invitations) to talk tends to convey, with the fewest words, the teacher's interest and reinforce the parent's communication. Of course, when a teacher wants to minimize a parent's verbosity, this strategy is contraindicated.

OTHER HELPFUL LEADS

The following are some phrases teachers may wish to use when they are fairly confident that their perceptions are accurate and the parent is receptive:

"You feel _____."
"It seems to you _____."
"From where you stand _____."
"As you see it _____."
"What you're saying is _____."
"I'm picking up that you _____."
"I really hear you saying that _____."

When the teacher is uncertain about her perception or senses that the parent might not be open to her observations, she might consider using the following phrases, which are more tentative:

"I'm not sure if I'm with you, but _____."
"What I guess I'm hearing is _____."
"Correct me if I'm wrong, but _____."
"This is what I think you are saying: _____."
"I'm not sure if I'm with you; do you mean _____?"
"Let me see if I'm with you; you _____."

Teachers should cautiously appraise what a parent may be communicating and consider most conclusions tentatively until they have been verified through the use of perception checks, which enable the parent to confirm or deny stated observations. Although we see many people who seemingly behave the same way in comparable situations, share attitudes and beliefs that vary little from person to person, and appear predictable in a number of ways, we must bear in mind the enormous complexity of human beings and how they are unique.

MICROTRAINING

In 1967, Dwight Allen developed an innovative approach to teacher training, which he called microteaching. Shortly thereafter, Allen Ivey at the University of Massachusetts adapted it to the training of counselors. Ivey's (1971) microcounseling model, which has influenced the training of counselors, has also been used to train teachers, paraprofessionals, children, teenagers, and college students; in fact, it can appropriately and easily be administered to anyone interested in developing effective interpersonal skills.

According to Ivey, microtraining is based on several assumptions:

1. It is possible to lessen the complexity of the interviewing process *by focusing on a single skill*. The objective of the interviewer is to master one skill at a time rather than to become competent in all areas simultaneously. It is this aspect of acquiring single, isolated skills, each taught separately, that significantly distinguishes this approach from other models.
2. Microtraining techniques provide important opportunities for *self-observation and self-confrontation*. An interviewer's role playing should be subject to immediate examination and critical evaluation by a supervisor by reviewing a videotape of the session with a supervisor, or by reviewing the videotape alone and conscientiously evaluating one's performance. What is important is that the practice session be examined *immediately* and be subject to *evaluation*.
3. Interviewers can learn from watching others' *social modeling* through videotaped demonstrations of the skills they wish to learn. Ivey has produced a series of microcounseling tapes that may be rented or purchased.
4. The skills taught in microcounseling cut across theoretical lines, because good, initial interpersonal skills are basic to all communication and therapeutic approaches.

The implementation of the microtraining model corresponds to the following steps, which are applied in a sequential fashion (adapted from Ivey, 1971, 1983).

1. The teacher receives instructions to enter a room where he will interview a role-played parent. Depending on the situation, the topic may or may not be defined. Similar instructions are given to the role-played parent, with the exception that she is told [that] she is about to be interviewed.
2. A 10- to 15-minute diagnostic session (with the teacher interviewing the "parent") is then videotaped.
3. The role-played parent leaves the room and completes an evaluation form. The form is available for the supervisory session with the teacher.

4. The teacher reads a written description of the specific skill to be learned in this session (e.g., Ivey, 1983; Egan, 1998). The supervisor talks with him about it (relating it to the content discussed in the manual).
5. Video models of an expert demonstrating the specific skill are shown. It is often helpful to have both a positive and a negative videotaped model of the skill to be learned.
6. The teacher is shown his initial interview and discusses it with his supervisor. He is asked to identify examples where he successfully engaged in or failed to apply the specific skill in question.
7. The supervisor and teacher review the skill together and plan for the next session.
8. The teacher reinterviews the same "parent" for 10 minutes.
9. Feedback and evaluation on the final session are made available to the teacher.

A scale such as the following may be used to evaluate the teacher's performance. The level of proficiency shown in the interview is rated on a 1- to 5-point scale.

	(1)	(2)	(3)	(4)	(5)	
Distant	1	2	3	4	5	Close
Open questions	1	2	3	4	5	Closed questions
Unfriendly	1	2	3	4	5	Friendly
Insecure	1	2	3	4	5	Secure
Confusing	1	2	3	4	5	Clear
Followed parent	1	2	3	4	5	Became tangential
Showed interest	1	2	3	4	5	Seemed disinterested
Rude	1	2	3	4	5	Polite
Nervous	1	2	3	4	5	Calm
Uncomfortable	1	2	3	4	5	Comfortable

You can add additional adjectives and make a rating scale that suits your purposes.

In a classroom or in a small group, such a scale may be completed by group members and given to the teacher. The teacher should review the returned scales and view the feedback as a constructive exercise. Such feedback should alert the teacher to areas of strengths and show where more practice is indicated. The areas that need work could be targeted in subsequent role playing.

ATTENDING BEHAVIOR

Ivey broke down into teachable units what he considered to be the essence of good listening, which he called "attending behavior." These units include eye contact, posture, and verbal following behavior. Ivey examined a number of studies supporting his contention that conscientious listening elicits uniformly positive feelings and behaviors on the part of others.

One approach to teaching attending behavior is to have the interviewer practice the direct *opposite* of the behavior to be learned. Then, to see the contrast between poor and proper behavior, he tries to do it correctly. The following exercise may be used to illustrate the concept:

1. Break up into pairs and decide (a) who will first play the role of the interviewer (teacher) and who will play the interviewee (parent); (b) the situation. You may refer to the critical incidents in Chapter 8 or make up other ones. Before the interview, it is generally helpful to give the teacher only a sketchy idea of the problem the parent intends to present.
2. For 3–4 minutes, engage in the *opposite* of the behavior (say, eye contact) that is under study.
3. After the 3–4 minutes, continue with the same topic but switch roles. Remember, *lack of eye contact* is still to be practiced.
4. Reverse roles again and for about the same amount of time (3–4 minutes) practice what you consider to be *appropriate* eye contact behavior.
5. Reverse roles again, so that both people have had an opportunity to practice the behavior properly.
6. Begin a discussion of the two conditions. For example, what was your reaction toward the interviewer when she used comfortable eye contact as opposed to when she did not? What general *feelings* were you aware of under the two conditions? What feelings about yourself did you realize?
7. After practicing both proper and improper eye contact, and after a debriefing session, move on to the next microunit and begin at item 1 again.

Below is a summary of Ivey's (1994) definitions of the three units that make up attending behavior. After reading the definitions, you should be ready to begin role playing.

1. *Posture.* The teacher should be physically relaxed and seated with natural posture but leaning slightly forward. If the teacher is comfortable, he is better able to listen to the person with whom he is talking. Also, if the teacher is relaxed physically, his posture and movements will be natural, thus increasing his own sense of well-being. This sense of comfortableness enables the teacher to better attend to and communicate with the parent. Egan (1994) describes the components of attending with the acronym SOLER.

S — sit squarely
O — open posture (not legs and arms crossed)
L — lean forward
E — eye contact
R — relax

2. *Eye contact.* The teacher should initiate and maintain eye contact with the parent. However, eye contact can be overdone. A varied use of eye contact is most effective, as staring fixedly or with undue intensity usually makes the parent uneasy. Heaton (1998) reminds us that eye contact, a learned behavior, is thus largely culturally determined. She notes, for example, that some people who have grown up in the inner city learn that it is dangerous to make eye contact.

3. *Verbal following behavior.* The final characteristic of good attending behavior is the teacher's use of comments that follow directly from what the parent is saying. By directing his comments and questions to what a parent just said, the teacher not only helps develop an area of discussion but also reinforces the parent's free expression, resulting in more spontaneity in their talk. Paraphrasing, which is discussed later in this chapter, resembles verbal following behavior but is a somewhat more sophisticated response.

Summary of Rules

The teacher's goal is to listen attentively and to communicate this attentiveness through relaxed posture, varied eye contact, and appropriate verbal responses.

1. Relax physically. Feel the presence of the chair as you are sitting on it. Let your posture be comfortable and your movements natural; for example, if you usually move and gesture a good deal, feel free to do so, but be cautions about excessive movements that may be disruptive during parent conferences.
2. Look at the person with whom you are talking.
3. Follow what the parents are saying by taking your cues from them. Do not jump from subject to subject or interrupt them, unless they become tangential. If you cannot think of anything to say, go back to something the parents said earlier in the conversation and ask them a question about that.

Murphy and Dillon (1998) offer the following exercise to illustrate nonattending: Have a conversation with a friend or school pal and, if possible, videotape the discussion. After talking for a few minutes, withdraw your attention by looking away or at your watch, cross your arms, or tap your feet. Notice what happens to the conversation. Ask your friend what it felt like when you stopped attending.

INTERPERSONAL PROCESS RECALL

Kagan, Holmes, and Kagan (1995) developed a process by which professionals may better understand their own inner experiencing in a helping relationship. A major objective of the model is to develop the ability to reflect on an interview shortly after it is over. Another objective is to develop the ability to sense and respond, if appropriate, to unverbalized perceptions and feelings present *during* an interview. Kagan et al.'s studies reveal that professional helpers have feelings and make observations during interviews of which they are aware at some level, but apparently, their awareness of more subtle aspects of an interview is not as acute as it might be.

The fact that teachers (and also parents) experience much more during a conference than is ever verbalized can be demonstrated by asking oneself, right after a conference, what was experienced during the meeting. Being keenly aware of one's feelings and thoughts is related to the notion of "immediacy." As Egan (1986) observes, "Once [the teacher] sees the richness of this unused material, he can learn to step back from the interview during the interview itself, see what the [parent] is doing, see what he himself is feeling and doing [or not doing], and use what he notices immediately" (p. 177).

Some time ago, Lister (1966) developed a concept of internal awareness and how it can help in interpersonal situations. (In reading the following quotation, the reader might substitute the word "teacher" for "counselor," and "parent" for "client.")

> Counselors have focused on clients' experiencing as a guide to their behavior during an interview. Most counselors feel that they can function more effectively when they know what is "going on" within another person. It seems that experiencing can also provide the counselor with a kind of "intrapersonal communication" which aids him in detecting and modifying within the immediate present subtle, moment-by-moment nuances of feelings within himself which disrupt his communication with his client. (p. 55)

Lister contends that outward signs of discomfort or threat are often preceded and accompanied by identifiable internal states. For example, when a teacher feels threatened (internal), her throat may tighten (external), causing a pinched, anxious tone in her voice; or she may become aware that tension in certain muscles was preceded by a feeling of anger.

Although being able to *respond* with immediacy during an interview is the primary goal of Kagan's interpersonal process recall (IPR) model, a teacher's *awareness* of her feelings toward a parent may be enough. To illustrate, a teacher may realize that a particular parent generates feelings of guilt and anger with comments such as "I wish you'd spend more time in class with my son" or "George always used to talk about Mrs. Grayson, his third-grade teacher, and how she used to make him feel like he had a second mother."

Instead of openly dealing with the parent's remarks or interpersonal style, which the teacher may not be able to alter anyway, her awareness of the effect the parent has on her (anger or guilt) gives her some significant data upon which to build a set of hypotheses about the parent. She may hypothesize that what she is experiencing probably is not unique to her and that others are treated in the same fashion and have similar responses. These insights may provide cues about the parent's child, for example, why other children tend to avoid him. The interpersonal style of the parent may reveal why the child responds with feelings of shame, guilt, and fear in relating to the teacher or other children. Conversely, a parent's openness and caring and the teacher's subsequent feelings of comfort in his presence help her understand why his child, who may be severely disabled, seems so much better adjusted psychologically than the other child.

The following process, which uses Kagan's IPR model during role playing, allows some general insights into the often-unexpressed feelings and perceptions of both teacher and parent. Each role play below has a parent and a teacher.

1. Divide the group or class into pairs.
2. Each pair engages in a 5-minute interview (you may wish to construct an interview, or use situations alluded to in other sections, or draw upon the critical incidents in Chapter 8).
3. At the end of the interview, each pair meets with another pair.
4. The role-played parent from pair *a* meets separately with the one from pair *b*. They help each other explore their feelings and perceptions about the interview, namely, what each parent thought and felt about himself, about the teacher, and about the interaction, but did not verbalize.
5. At the same time, the two persons who role-played teachers meet and do the same thing.
6. After about 10 minutes, all four members meet together. The two members of pair *b* help the two members from pair *a* share thoughts and feelings that were not verbalized.
7. The process outlined in item 6 is repeated, with pair *a* helping pair *b*.
8. Discuss the process and what you learned from the exercise in the larger group class.

PARAPHRASING

Paraphrasing is the technique that constitutes the core of good interviewing because it captures the essence of understanding: *empathy*. Good listening and attending are its necessary prerequisites.

Paraphrases serve three purposes: (1) to convey to the parent that the teacher is trying to understand what is being said; (2) to crystallize parent's comments by making them more concise, thus giving better direction to the interview; and (3) to check the accuracy of the teacher's perceptions.

One can distinguish paraphrasing from simple restatement:

PARENT: I don't know about him. One moment he's nice as can be, and the next minute he is a real jerk.

TEACHER 1: He's a real jerk. [Restatement]

TEACHER 2: He's pretty inconsistent, then. [Paraphrase]

or:

TEACHER 3: His inconsistent behavior makes it difficult to trust him. [Paraphrase]

Paraphrases, then, go beyond restatements and tend to capture the core of what someone is saying (Heaton, 1998).

Brammer (1973) breaks down paraphrases into feeling and content. *Content* paraphrasing repeats in fewer and fresher words the essential *ideas* of another person. It is used to clarify ideas that the parent may be expressing with some difficulty. In paraphrasing, the teacher tries to find the essence of what is being said rather than just restating the words.

Two examples of *content* paraphrases follow:

PARENT: Sometimes Ron seems close to us and affectionate and at other times he is distant and preoccupied.

TEACHER: He tends to move in and out of your relationship with him. His behavior can be puzzling to you sometimes.

An example of a restatement that would not be considered a poor response might be:

TEACHER: Sometimes Ron is close to you and at other times more distant.

This paraphrase goes beyond simple restatement by focusing on the *relationship* between Ron and his parents and not just on Ron's behavior. It also reflects what must be a confusing situation for Ron's parents ("His behavior can be kind of puzzling").

PARENT: Every time I come here to talk with you, I feel like a burden . . . as if you have other things you have to do.

TEACHER: You seem to be saying to me that I give signals that tell you that I would rather be doing something else than talking with you. Can you tell me a little more about this so that I can better understand?

This paraphrase focuses on possible cues the parent is picking up from the teacher's behavior. It is important to recognize that the parent may feel like a burden to most people; thus, her comment has more to do with how she feels about herself than about her relationship with the teacher. Such a comment from a parent may give the teacher some insight into her own unrecognized behavior, or it may suggest that she is dealing with a parent who is exceptionally sensitive to the slightest indication of rejection. Only additional conversation will reveal whether the teacher should take a closer look at her own nonverbal cues or proceed gingerly with a parent who is prone to misinterpret her actions. In the previous paraphrase, the teacher also asks the parent to elaborate on his response to allow her to understand him fully.

A *feeling* paraphrase involves expressing in fresh words the essential *feelings*, stated or strongly implied, of the parent. The purpose of reflecting feelings is to focus on emotions rather than content, and to bring vaguely expressed emotions into clearer focus.

To help others with their feelings, one must understand one's own. For reasons too complex to discuss at length here, some people are cut off from their emotional life, having learned early, for example, that feelings lead to bad consequences or to a loss of control. The result probably is suppression, a conscious defense mechanism that keeps unpleasant events, thoughts, feelings, and so on, below one's awareness yet not completely inaccessible. Teachers and counselors who chronically suppress their feelings tend to discourage the affective expressions of persons they are in a position to help. If feelings are considered dangerous, they are dangerous whether expressed by oneself or by others.

Most authors believe that to help others clarify their feelings, one must understand his or her own feelings. Prospective helpers can better understand how their feelings manifest themselves by reflecting on the concomitants of certain emotions. To illustrate: "When I feel *accepted*, I feel warm inside / feel safe / feel free to be myself." "When I feel *scared*, I feel like running away / feel vulnerable / feel like crying."

In a small group, each person can discuss the relationship between a feeling (e.g., fear) and how it is manifested (e.g., feeling vulnerable). It is important to keep in mind that feelings are not bad. They are human and normal, and provide cues to subsequent behavior. Some common feelings are as follows:

1. Anger—wanting to say something mean
2. Anxiety—"I feel inadequate whenever Dr. Collins comes in to meet with me about his son, Timothy."

3. Boredom
4. Competitiveness
5. Confusion
6. Defensiveness
7. Frustration
8. Guilt
9. Hurt
10. Loneliness
11. Love or warmth
12. Rejection
13. Confidence

A review of the two incidents presented earlier suggests that the following *feelings* may be inferred from the parents' comments:

PARENT: Sometimes Ron seems close to us and affectionate, and at other times he seems distant and preoccupied. [*Possible feelings:* confusion, upset, disappointment, frustration, ambivalence, manipulation.]

PARENT: Every time I come here to talk with you, I feel like a burden, as if you have other things you have to do. [*Possible feelings:* rejection, hurt, anger, inferiority.]

A *feeling* paraphrase of the comments by the parent who feels like a burden might be as follows:

TEACHER: I think you're telling me that you feel as if you are not important [rejected, hurt] and therefore feel like you're bothering me [a burden]. It's almost as if I don't care to talk with you.

Unless the relationship with a parent is fairly close, teachers should allude to feelings indirectly (e.g., "you are not important") rather than exposing them directly by using words such as "hurt" or "rejection." Some words or phrases may cut too deeply when a parent is not accustomed to relating to a teacher in a more intimate fashion.

Feeling paraphrases must be used judiciously. They challenge a teacher's sense of timing and judgment more than any other response. When a parent is in trouble, teachers are there to be supportive, not to uncover deep feelings best dealt with by a trained psychotherapist.

TIMING

Timing in an interview is a combination of experience and good judgment. Responses to parents are based on a teacher's generalized knowledge of people as well as knowledge of the specific situation and parent. For example, if a parent is anxious and excessively concerned about her son's upcoming surgery, the teacher would certainly not initiate a discussion of the son's academic progress.

Losen and Diament (1978) equate timing in a parent conference with the timing used in playing chess, where one wishes to make initial moves that afford the greatest latitude or number of alternatives for later courses of action. And Heaton (1998) observes that "when we give an explanation (or ask a question) prematurely, it bounces off, makes the client (parent) defensive or ruptures rapport. If it is given too late, we're inefficient. In other words, timing is crucial" (p. 139).

Some researchers believe that timing in interpersonal situations can make the difference between the acceptance or rejection of an opinion or idea. When parents are in a projecting (blaming others) mood, simple listening and responding (paraphrasing) may be the best course of action. When the same parents become more accepting of their child's disability and appear ready to allow their child to engage in extended classroom activities, the teacher should include ideas and suggestions to which the parents are now responsive. Conversely, parents who are coping well and wish to learn a specific teaching strategy to work more productively with their child at home require a more active relationship with the teacher and less of a supportive one.

Teachers concerned about proper timing may become excessively self-conscious, especially beginners. Even though concerning oneself with proper timing may be inhibiting in some respects, it does serve notice to teachers that an utterance may be far more effective at one point in a relationship than at another. The self-consciousness decreases as teachers learn to trust their own intuitive sense of timing. Those who seem to have problems with timing, however, need good supervision.

HOW AND WHEN TO BE SUPPORTIVE

One way to get a perspective on supportive responses is to consider their opposites: probing, interpreting, advising, cajoling, lecturing, or judging. In contrast, supportive comments inform parents that teachers understand their predicament and will not abandon them during trying periods. Supportive statements often implicitly encourage someone who is troubled to continue in the face of adversity. Reassurance, a component of support, reassures parents that the situation with which they are struggling has an attainable goal.

In using supportive responses, the teacher should have determined that the parent is undergoing a concern of some magnitude or a crisis that requires some type of support. Also note that in the following examples, a paraphrase precedes a supportive comment.

PARENT: I don't know what I'm going to do. Alice has become so moody and hard to deal with that I find it more and more difficult to be nice to her.

TEACHER: I hear you saying that Alice's moodiness seems to be making it harder to interact with her in a positive way. [Paraphrase] I can sense your frustration in coming to grips with the situation. It must be difficult for you. [Supportive statement]

PARENT: We learned last week from our pediatrician that what we were afraid of these past few years is true. Dr. Ferguson told us that Tommy will never be able to walk.

TEACHER: That must have been quite a blow to have your worst fears confirmed. [Paraphrase] I feel badly that the news wasn't more positive, but over time, I feel certain that some of the things that Tommy can do will stand out more than the things he can't do. [Supportive statement]

These responses contain definite elements of reassurance. However, in the example in which the parent received bad news from Dr. Ferguson, the teacher should beware of cutting short a period of mourning that the parent needs to negotiate. If the parent appears to accept the support and reassurance, the teacher should continue to provide it; if not, he should revert to something like the initial supportive reflection ("That must have been quite a blow to have your worst fears confirmed").

PARENT: As you know, Timmy will be going to a new school next year. We are worried that he will not continue to get the kind of education and attention he has gotten here.

TEACHER: I can sense your concern and can appreciate your feelings of uneasiness in facing a new and unknown situation. Several other parents who faced similar situations told me that their youngster eased into the new school very nicely and that they were pleased that the move didn't hamper their child's learning.

In general, try to remain supportive without being suffocating: for example, "Don't worry, Mrs. Wilson, I know everything will be OK, so you need not worry about a thing." In your quest to be helpful, be wary of making statements that only someone in another profession (e.g., medicine) can make. For example, in one of the earlier situations, a teacher might comment: "I wouldn't take Dr. Ferguson's diagnosis seriously. I've seen boys with Tommy's condition before, and sooner or later they begin to walk." Such remarks, said more to ease the teacher's anxiety (by lessening the parent's grief) than to be of genuine help, are misleading rather than supportive.

Do not confuse sympathy with support. Support conveys understanding and caring, whereas sympathy connotes pity. Few of us tolerate the condescending communication of sympathy from another.

Give some thought to how you would feel or react as a recipient of the following supportive and sympathetic responses:

1. "I sense that you are concerned about Tommy's progress in school." [Supportive]
   "It must be terrible to always be anxious about how Tommy is doing in school." [Sympathetic]
2. "That must have been quite a blow to have your worst fears confirmed." [Supportive]
   "I really feel sorry for people when they get such tragic news." [Sympathetic]
3. "Hearing that from your husband must have hurt." [Supportive]
   "Oh, you poor thing. It's a pity that a good person like you has to tolerate such language from her husband." [Sympathetic]

HOW AND WHEN TO BE ASSERTIVE AND FIRM

There are instances in our personal lives when it is necessary to be firm. A roommate's tendency to shirk responsibility for cleaning up, buying the groceries, and helping with the finances requires that we eventually confront the situation that is generating anger. A discussion with the roommate is in order. Perhaps in the roommate's view, the existing situation is not subject to change. In such an instance, we may wish to discuss the limits within which one is willing to continue to share the apartment; that is, we are *asserting* our right as an equal partner in the shared apartment.

The words "firm," "assertive," and "confrontive" are often used to convey essentially the same notion: displeasure with an existing situation (recognition of a feeling), the desire to openly discuss it (being confrontive or assertive), and the intention to set limits should the discussion fail to achieve a mutually acceptable conclusion.

On occasion, teachers find it necessary to confront a situation of long standing. Consider, for example, the parent who volunteers as an aide in the classroom. Most teachers would welcome some help in the classroom, but within limits. This hypothetical parent, because of her compulsive or monopolizing manner, has a tendency to take over. She initiates activity without the teacher's consent or approval and, in her zeal to be helpful, has lost her perspective on the role of a volunteer. When the aide becomes more of a burden than an asset, the teacher needs to confront the situation by pointing out the role of both teacher and aide in the classroom. The aide, however, should be allowed to express her views and her reaction to the teacher's confrontation. If she accepts the teacher's observations, then the teacher can outline the ways in which the two parties may complement each other in the classroom. A parent who is totally insensitive to her role may require a firmer response:

> "I very much appreciate your desire to be helpful to me in the classroom, but I feel that I work best when I can tell you how you might be able to help when you are here. If you feel comfortable with this, I would very much welcome your continued help, but if you feel too constrained by what I am suggesting, then I would ask that you reconsider working with me."

Fortunately, such firmness is generally unnecessary, but when it is required, it is better to be assertive than to internalize one's anger and growing sense of frustration.

We have all been in situations where an assertive response on our part would have been gratifying, but we often withdraw because of some felt risk. Therefore, being assertive is considerably easier to talk about than to implement.

Consider the following incidents that commonly arise in daily living and require some type of assertive response.

1. A friend or colleague that you are very fond of has a habit of
   _____ [think of a real and annoying habit]. The habit is so annoying that you feel you have to discuss [with your friend] the
   effect it has on you.
2. You feel that your supervisor consistently treats you in a condescending manner. You believe that this behavior is unwar-
   ranted and you plan to discuss it at your next conference.
3. You have been treated shabbily and in a demeaning manner by
   a sales clerk. You feel justifiably angry and you are about ready
   to assert yourself in this situation.

Consider what you would say in the following parent–teacher situations that require an assertive or firm response from you (in each instance, assume that the situation requires an assertive response):

• At every conference the parent makes an issue of the fact that
you are using inappropriate materials for your students. Because you
are conscientious, you sought feedback from your peers and re-
searched the materials extensively. You even experimented with other
materials and are now convinced that those you selected are the most
appropriate.

• A parent insists that you are the only one who can help him
with some serious personal problems. You have tried subtly to tell the
parent you are not trained to help him with these problems, but to no
avail.

• The parent continually moans about the lack of progress her
child has made. You feel strongly that the child needs to work on his
deficiencies outside of class to reinforce gains made in class. The parent, however, refuses to spend any time working on academics with
her child and feels that such activity should remain in the classroom.

• Whenever a father and mother meet with you for a conference,
they begin to fight with each other, revealing marital problems that
you feel can be dealt with effectively by a professional counselor. You
have witnessed this situation a few times now and have been reluctant
to suggest marital counseling; now, you have come to the conclusion
that you will deal with this issue at the next conference.

It is crucial to recognize some differences between assertive responses (expressing oneself appropriately) and aggressive responses
(unbridled release). Assertive responses:

1. Increase feelings of self-worth as well as self-worth of others.
2. Express what one feels and thinks and encourage others to do so; usually convey friendly, affectionate, nonanxious feelings.
3. Usually achieve goals and encourage others to achieve their goals.
4. Make one feel less anxious and more competent; others feel comfortable and at ease in expressing themselves.
5. Generate feelings on part of others that one is not punitive and is more likely to rationally evaluate situations.
6. In response to unreasonable requests one politely refuses and explains reasons. (Alberti & Emmons, 1970, p. 23)

In contrast, aggressive responses:

1. Increase self-worth but deny worth of others; others feel disparaged and even humiliated.
2. Express what one feels and thinks but deny opportunity for such expression by others.
3. Achieve goals by downgrading others; thus others usually do not achieve goals.
4. Depreciate others so that they feel hurt, defensive, and incompetent.
5. In response to an unreasonable request one tends to refuse angrily, which makes others either defensive or angry. (Alberti & Emmons, 1970, p. 24)

THE USE OF QUESTIONS

It is a foregone conclusion that questions constitute a large portion of an interview—or is it? Benjamin (1987) believes that interviewers (teachers) ask too many meaningless questions, and ones an interviewee (parents) cannot possibly answer. Questions are often posed that actually confuse or interrupt the interviewee (parent) or that the interviewer (teacher) doesn't want answered, resulting in responses he does not hear. By asking questions and getting answers, asking more questions and getting more answers, a teacher may be setting up a pattern from which neither parent nor teacher can be extricated.

The ultimate test for asking a question may be stated thusly: "Will the question I am about to ask further or inhibit the flow of the interview?" In using questions, Benjamin (1987, p. 135) suggests:

1. We should be aware of the fact that we are asking questions.
2. We should challenge the questions we are about to ask and weigh carefully the desirability of asking them.
3. We should examine carefully the various sorts of questions available to us and the types of questions we personally tend to use.
4. We should consider alternatives to the asking of questions.
5. We should become sensitive to the questions the interviewee is asking, whether he is asking them outright or not.

First, let us examine the types of questions available to us.

Open versus Closed Questions

According to Benjamin (1987), *open* questions tend to be broad; allow the interviewee full scope; widen his perceptual field; solicit views, opinions, thoughts, and feelings; widen and deepen the contact. For example:

> "Jerry appears to be quite active these days. He seems to be at an age where there is much to stimulate him. What do you think?"
> "You don't seem to be your usual self today. Anything happen? Some kids really like school and others are turned off by it. How do you think Jerry feels about school?"

In contrast, *closed* questions are narrow, limit the respondent to a specific answer, curtail the perceptual field, demand cold facts only, and circumscribe the contact. For example:

> "How old is Jerry?"
> "When is he going to camp?"
> "Does Amy seem to like school?"

Another type of *closed* question includes the answer, or at least strongly implies that the respondent agree:

> "Isn't it obvious that Karen doesn't care about the kids she teaches?"
> "Everyone knows that Mr. and Mrs. Goldberg are real pains, isn't that so?"
> "There's no question that this school is the worst one to teach in, right?"

This type of questioning does not allow parents to indicate alternate views.

Direct versus Indirect Questions

Direct questions are obvious queries, whereas indirect questions inquire without seeming to do so and are more open. The latter do not end in a question mark, yet it is evident that a question is being asked.

> *Direct:* "Isn't it rough working with such unmotivated kids?"
> *Indirect:* "It must be rough working with kids who have trouble motivating themselves."
> *Direct:* "How do you like your new teaching job?"
> *Indirect:* "I wonder how the new teaching job seems to you."
> *Direct:* "What do you think of the new token economy system we're using?"
> *Indirect:* "You must have some thoughts about our new token economy system."
> *Direct:* "How does it feel to be in your new school?"
> *Indirect:* "I'd sure like to know how you feel about your new school."

Even more than open questions, indirect questions allow for a variety of responses.

Double Questions

Double questions limit the parent to one of two choices. Some examples follow:

> "Do you want to set up an appointment for 2 or 3 weeks?"
> "Would you like to have coffee or tea?"
> "Do you want Jimmy to be a teacher or social worker?"
> "Do you want to sit near Celeste or Irma?"

Simple double questions like these curtail a parent's perceptual field and response and should be avoided *when other alternatives exist.* Of course, where only two possibilities are available, one should not imply that more options exist.

Examples of more elaborate *double questions*, which tend to confuse, are as follows:

"Have we covered everything we wanted to today, and what do
you think about scheduling an appointment for our next conference?"

"Is Jimmy more controllable now at home, and how is his toilet
training coming along?"

"Did you get a chance to see an orthopedic surgeon about Karen's
hip, and what did the eye doctor say about her vision?"

A simple solution to this problem is to ask each question singly.

"Why" Questions

To Benjamin (1987) "why" questions are the most useless and potentially destructive type because they often connote disapproval or displeasure. Thus, whenever someone hears the word "why," he may feel
the need to defend herself, to withdraw and avoid the situation, or to
take the offensive. However, this type of reaction is generally less
likely when rapport between two people is favorable, that is, when
trust and respect are present.

It is interesting to note that, for children, the word "why" has a
different meaning than it has for adults. Children often ask "why"
questions as a key to unlock the world about them; thus for them,
"why" is used to gain information.

In adult-to-adult relationships, "why" is too often perceived as
"Don't do that" or "You ought to be ashamed." As a result, a parent
may withdraw into himself, become angry, or rationalize, and consequently distance himself from the teacher. Rather than feeling free to
explore and experience, the parent will feel threatened and resort to
defending himself.

The following are some examples of "why" questions that often
are perceived negatively. Discuss in your group or think privately of
what your feelings would be as a recipient of these questions:

"Why don't you have your Halloween bulletin boards in black
and orange?"

"Why are you late to our conference today?"

"Why doesn't Bruce wear warmer clothing during the winter
months?"

"Why doesn't Rita read better since we discussed her home reading program?"

By asking these kinds of questions in a more indirect way, they can be framed so that they will have less bite.

> "I noticed that Bruce seems to be cold during class and I was wondering if there might be something he could wear so that he would feel more comfortable."
> "I noticed that Rita hasn't improved her reading very much since our last conference. I wonder what we could do that would motivate her to read more often."
> "You must have run into that terrible downtown traffic on your way here."

During the next few weeks, become aware of the *types of questions* you tend to ask and the circumstances under which you ask them. You might also develop a more acute awareness of your response (internal and verbal) to questions that are posed to you (especially "why" questions), as well as the types of questions people around you tend to ask.

INTERPRETATION: PROS AND CONS

In counseling, the technique of interpreting behavior or feelings has met with a mixed response. Interpretation is the hallmark of Freudian-oriented counseling—which is not to say that it is the sum and substance of Freud's theory, but interpretive responses constitute the basic therapeutic technique. In contrast, proponents of person-centered counseling (developed by Carl Rogers) eschew interpretation and believe that improved relationships and positive personality growth are achieved under the guidance of an empathic, warm, and genuine professional. Thus, insights are made by the client.

Interpretations made by a counselor (or teacher) convey his perceptions, not the client's (or parents); therefore, their value as a facilitative technique in building rapport is limited. Some researchers argue that reflections, summarizations, and paraphrases are indeed interpretations, but more subtle ones. Be that as it may, the purpose of this section is to show how interpretation may be of practical help in some situations and useless or even destructive in others.

Interpretation serves the function of providing information without mistakes or distortion. For example, when a parent confers about her child's test scores, the teacher will want to interpret them accurately. Interpretation often lessens the parent's sense of ambiguity.

> "Sure, Mr. Compomizzi, I'd be happy to go over Jimmy's reading test results with you. On the vocabulary section, he scored _____ in the _____ percentile, meaning that _____ % scored above and _____ % scored below Jimmy. On the comprehension section of the test, he scored _____, again telling us that _____ % did better than Jimmy, compared to thousands of others who took the test and scored lower. In general, his test scores at this point tend to indicate that he would have difficulty in a straight academic program in school. At this point I'd be interested in your observations and thoughts. Any questions come to mind?"

Sometimes, when parents are at a complete loss, for example, about their child's behavior they may come to the teacher for help. Should the teacher feel that her perspective can be of assistance, she could interpret what she believes is causing the child's behavior, but in a way that allows parents to respond to her observations:

> "It's quite possible that Amy is acting up these days because of the birth of her baby brother. It is not unusual for a child to behave differently when she realizes that she won't get as much attention as she used to and feels left out to a certain extent. What do you think, Mr. Phillips? Does this make sense to you?"

Interpretations of behavior can be of immense value to a parent, but they also have a dangerous aspect. People often resent having their feelings and behavior interpreted. For example, how would you feel if a teacher you did not know well commented:

> "Boy, you sure do let quiet, shy Joan have it full blast. I think the reason you're so harsh with her is because she reminds you of your mother's introverted behavior that you hated. In a way, it's like striking back at your mother through Joan."
>
> "Now I understand why Jeff is so emotionally disturbed. It's hard for a child to feel secure in a home like yours, where everyone is yelling and blaming each other for things."
>
> "Your anxiety about George's lack of progress is unfounded. What is happening is that you're putting your own need to

achieve on your son, and by doing that, you're placing undue pressure on him and making him a nervous wreck."

Although sometimes accurate, such interpretations almost always generate anger and defensive responses. "Anxiety," as used here, is an emotionally laden term and should generally be avoided unless parents use it to refer to themselves. To declare that parents' feelings are "unfounded" makes them feel silly or stupid in having them. Fears and anxieties are not necessarily based on obvious events; some people can be as fearful of a friendly crowd as others are of a deadly snake. By starting a sentence, "What is happening is . . . ", the teacher is implying that her word is above question. Interpreting a parent's own need to achieve (although it may be correct) can certainly make him feel uncomfortable for a variety of reasons—not the least of which is the fact that he is not meeting with the teacher for personal psychotherapy. To remark that the parent is putting a great deal of pressure on his son can only lead to feelings of guilt—feelings that the parent may already experience. Finally, suggesting that the son is a "nervous wreck" either reinforces or arouses in the parent the possibility that the boy has a psychiatric problem.

All in all, these responses are most destructive. By *reflecting* instead of interpreting material the parent has already provided, a teacher can facilitate awareness without generating guilt, resentment, anger, and lowered self-esteem. For example:

> "I hear you saying that you have a tendency to be hard on yourself and you're wondering whether you might also be hard on George."

The teacher is paraphrasing something to which the parent, in his own words, has alluded; the *core meaning* is reflected back.

HOME CONFERENCES

Teachers often do not have time to make frequent home visits; however, home visits by teachers are increasingly more common (Shea & Bauer, 1991). There are times when teachers should seriously consider such conferences; in fact, the practice is standard in many preschool and special education programs. As noted in Chapter 5, in conducting home conferences, keep the following issues in mind:

1. Do not schedule such a meeting until you have proposed it to the parents.
2. Never drop by for an unannounced visit.
3. Be on time. Parents may not be prepared for an early arrival, and they would most likely resent awaiting the arrival of a teacher who is significantly late.
4. To the extent possible, honor the time schedule you initially established with the parents.
5. Don't overdress or wear the jeans that you wear to a ball game. The clothes you normally wear in class should suffice.
6. Both parents should have a general sense of the purpose of the visit.
7. Upon arrival, talk informally with the parents and child for a few minutes to establish a friendly tone.
8. Refusing to eat or drink what parents offer may hurt their feelings. If you do not wish to indulge, mention having eaten shortly before the visit. It is customary to be offered some repast when visiting in someone's home, and it is generally considered disrespectful to refuse. Rapport tends to be enhanced when a teacher accepts an offer of food or drink.
9. Try not to cancel a home visit. Parents spend a considerable amount of physical and mental energy preparing for it. A cancellation can hurt morale, especially for the heretofore uncooperative parents who are making an effort to establish a relationship with the teacher. However, sometimes, cancellations are simply unavoidable.
10. Be prepared for distractions. Children running and shouting, phone calls, and visitors dropping by may interrupt the conference. Although you hope that the parents provide a distraction-free conference, some situations are beyond your control. You are now in the parents' territory. For most parents, there will be other, distraction-free conferences at school, where the teacher can discuss more serious matters.

There may be circumstances when the teacher may want to consider bringing another school professional along (e.g., social worker, school nurse) if he expects to broach topics that may cause conflict, or if there is a history of strained home–school relationships (Turnbull & Turnbull, 1986). A colleague can serve as a support person or a mediator in the event of a serious disagreement.

The home visit is best used to help the teacher establish or continue rapport with parents and become more knowledgeable about the family. There are definite advantages to home visits, but there are also a few drawbacks: They are time-consuming and sometimes inconvenient for both parties and, as noted earlier, parents and teachers need to plan for the visit (Shea & Bauer, 1991).

REFERRALS

A number of times thus far in this volume, I have recommended that the teacher refer the parent to other professionals for help when appropriate. Some professionals (e.g., physician, social worker) make referrals routinely. However, because parents may be less likely to expect a referral from a teacher, the process becomes somewhat delicate. Referrals for psychological reasons are particularly sensitive, as both parties must deal with what such a referral implies.

Referrals are made for a variety of reasons. Hornby (1995) discusses the value of an appropriate referral for children who have suffered a major loss, such as divorce, or the death of a parent or other central family member. More challenging for the teacher are those referrals that involve conflicts within the family, such as problems or disagreements regarding the child with a disability, abuse in the family, perhaps aided by substance abuse, or intractable stress. To illustrate how a referral might be offered, a teacher might make the following comment after noting the conflicts generated by family stress during the Gibbons conference:

> "I've noticed that in the last two meetings, both of you seem to be experiencing a considerable amount of stress. I know how draining chronic stress can be on a family and how it gets in the way of family goals. I wonder if you have thought about visiting a psychologist who is an expert at helping families cope with stressful situations? I know of some resources that can be helpful if you would like to hear about them."

Although the teacher is not a qualified psychological counselor, professional helpers, like teachers, possessing solid, basic conferencing skills, can deal effectively with transitory problems. In this regard, it would be helpful if teachers learned to be less fearful of parents' emotions and problems. In most cases, just being a supportive listener is all that is required. Because of their status in the community and their contacts with parents and their children, teachers often are in an excellent position to make referrals. Numerous agencies, and the like, listed in the Appendix, may prove to be helpful to teachers. It is useful to augment this list with other information that is particularly relevant to the teachers' community.

Teachers should be sure the community has the necessary resources to accomplish the goals of the referral. Introducing the subject to a parent requires discretion and a warm, caring manner. The teacher should make clear and communicate unambiguously the justification for the referral to the parent, such as in the previous example.

Counseling for significant personal or family problems can be a long-term process if positive and lasting effects are to be obtained. Thus, the teacher should not be impatient to see problems diminish or vanish but should remain supportive of the parents' efforts to seek help and attempt change no matter how long it takes or how difficult the process.

SELF-HELP ORGANIZATIONS

Although peer self-help groups are currently enjoying enormous popularity, Konopka (1972) points out that support groups parallel the history of social services as they evolved within a changing society. The older social services, which distinguished sharply between the giver and receiver, were generally referred to as philanthropy. As people moved from farm to city and from foreign countries to the United States, mutual self-help groups sprang up to meet the ever-increasing need for aid, identity, and support. For example, there were the brotherhoods that developed their own centers, such as the Jewish Community Centers and settlement houses for various nationalities. These groups were initially conceived and run by outsiders, but they gradually took on their own responsibilities as they evolved.

"Self-help groups" can be defined as a human-service-oriented voluntary associations made up of individuals who share a problem or life circumstance and who meet to resolve or cope with the problem through their mutual efforts (Borkman, 1976, cited in Marsh, 1992). There are a number of potential benefits in membership, such as discovering that one is not struggling alone; finding a sense of belonging; receiving assistance that is affordable and nonstigmatizing, long-term support, a vehicle for empowerment, and a place to get information; and finding opportunities to develop skills and coping mechanisms (Lieberman, 1990; Seligman, 1993). Both clinical and data-based evidence indicate that support groups for families who have a member with a disability are helpful (Hornby, 1994; Meyer & Vadasy, 1994).

One parent, quoted in Marsh (1992), had the following view of the support group she attended:

> "Meeting other mothers with similar experiences was wonderful. As much as we love our handicapped children, it was such an eye-opener to learn that other mothers had intense feelings at times of guilt, anger toward the child, resentment toward an abnormal lifestyle, and other negative feelings. I thought I was the only one that still felt this way after so many years. I left the meetings uplifted that my feelings were quite typical and really normal considering what our family has gone through." (p. 195)

Self-help groups were, and to some extent still are, characterized by a desire for citizen action to improve ones lot or to help improve that of others. Marsh (1992) estimates that there are more than 500,000 self-help groups in the United States. These groups exist for many populations and meet a variety of needs not addressed by professional services.

In an effort to provide much needed help to parents of exceptional children in the Lexington, Kentucky area, Project Cope was born, and the Parent Club was formed as an outgrowth of group counseling under its auspices. The goals, operations, and functions of the Parent Club, as described by Taylor (1976), parallel to a large extent other parental self-help groups that currently exist. The club has three primary objectives: (1) to provide social activities, (2) to provide educational opportunities through speakers in various professional fields, and (3) to develop projects to increase parents' identity as a group and provide some avenue for self-awareness and leadership for their children. The Parent Club has been instrumental in establishing a state bureau of special education and a law permitting public schools to purchase services from private agencies. It is also active in various fund-raising projects.

In a more general sense, self-help organizations evolve as a consequence of the perceived needs of parents for mutual support, inspiration, education, and social action. Self-help groups may also be of practical assistance, by providing babysitting arrangements and transportation for members. Because such organizations can be an enormous help to parents of children with disabilities, it would be most advantageous for teachers to be aware of the ones that exist in their community. Parent-to-parent groups, as well as those for fathers and siblings, are available in many communities.

BIBLIOTHERAPY

Bibliotherapy is a fancy word for a rather simple yet helpful strategy—the use of reading material to help someone better understand a condition or situation, or to provide support, encouragement, and a sense of universality (a feeling that others have similar problems). Parents of children with disabilities, especially those who like to read and/or desire information about their child's condition, can benefit from the judicious referral to pertinent reading material. Some parents, as well as children, also achieve insights and encouragement by reading biographies and classical literature involving a disability. It is helpful to keep in mind that although for some people such books are inspiring, for others they may symbolize unattainable achievements. Reading material can give hope and provide meaning to the lives of parents, siblings, and the child with a disability (Peterson & Nisenholz, 1987).

Written sources may also inform parents of legislation related to their child's exceptionality, where needed services may be sought, as well as the exact nature of these services, or how to deal effectively with a particular situation (e.g., toilet training, dressing, and undressing).

Although bibliotherapy is generally viewed in a positive fashion, some books may be a mixed blessing. They can sometimes be so brief as to be misleading, include too much too soon, or are written from the point of view of a specific philosophy that may conflict with parents' plans for a particular child.

Bibliotherapy does not simplify a professional's responsibilities. Teachers should be familiar with published material so that they can recommend appropriate selections. Recommended readings should include materials that are objective, rather than misleading and biased, and compatible with the goals parents wish to achieve. The selection of appropriate reading materials may help parents feel less alone and contribute to their general knowledge about their concerns.

In the Appendix, a list of available readings is grouped into specific categories. In order to make appropriate referrals to the readings, teachers should be knowledgeable about their content and quality. It is therefore recommended that teachers keep apprised of new articles, books, and journals that may be of value to parents. Finally, rather than monitor what a parent reads, it is the task of the teacher to make referrals to appropriate sources when it seems advisable, or when a parent requests it. If possible, it is helpful if teachers make themselves available to discuss articles or books. Some reading materials require interpretation or elaboration by a professional; others stimulate thoughts and ideas that parents may wish to share with their child's teacher.

7

The Individualized Education Program Conference

The collaboration of parents and teachers was formalized by the passage of key legislation. Prior to such legislative efforts, parent conferences were a haphazard affair. School personnel who voiced support for collaboration between families and schools conducted conferences in an informal, unstructured manner, whereas teachers who felt that such conferences constituted an unnecessary activity, or felt burdened by other school-related tasks, simply did not have them. As a result, some parents felt that they were partners in their child's education, while others believed that it was solely the school's responsibility to make educational decisions on behalf of their children.

Turnbull and Turnbull (1986) contend that there are three major reasons why the federal government decided that it is appropriate to get involved in the education of children with disabilities. First, schools had historically excluded those children from any education. Children who were not mobile or toilet trained, who evidenced behavioral problems or were deemed unable to profit from existing educational programs, were excluded. When the Education for All Handicapped Children Act was enacted in 1974, it was discovered that one million children with disabilities were not receiving any education.

Second, nearly half of the children with disabilities enrolled in some sort of educational program were not receiving an *appropriate* education. The notion of an appropriate education is discussed in more detail shortly. Third, schools were employing assessment procedures (intelligence or psychological tests) inappropriately.

> For example, a child who speaks only Spanish might have been given a test in English; a child with a learning disability might have been required to take a test in the same way and in the same period of time as children who have no disabilities; poor Black children might have been asked questions that are appropriate only for white middle-class children; or a child with cerebral palsy might be asked to write answers to a test when she has so little manual dexterity that she cannot hold a pencil. (Turnbull & Turnbull, 1986, p. 167)

There were a number of reasons that schools excluded children with disabilities. First, the cost of educating these children was generally higher than the cost of educating nondisabled children. Second, children with disabilities had little political influence in schools or in the government. Third, educators believed that children with disabilities could not learn fast enough to profit from an education. The final reason, fueled by inaccurate notions and prejudicial thinking, was that these children were not regarded as worthy of an education (Turnbull & Turnbull, 1986).

LEGISLATIVE INITIATIVES

What legislative mandates have led to the current focus on Individualized Education Program (IEP) conferences that is now a required component of a child's educational experience? Public Law 89-750, the Education of the Handicapped Act, which was passed in 1966, provided federal grants to help states initiate, expand, and improve special education. With a particular emphasis on severe disabilities, the Rehabilitation Act of 1973 proposed that vocational services be provided to persons with disabilities. The Rehabilitation Act had as its chief goal planning and preparing gainful employment for persons with disabilities. Section 504 of the Rehabilitation Act prohibited employment discrimination on the basis of physical, cognitive, or sensory disabilities (Alper et al., 1994). Employers who received governmental monies and did not adhere to Section 504 guidelines could be penalized. Section 504 also protects students with disabilities in school settings even if they do not have an IEP (F. Prezant, personal communication, June 15, 1999). The most outward manifestation of the Rehabilitation Act of 1973 and the subsequent Americans with Disabilities Act was the installation of curb cuts, wider doorways, grab bars, ramps, and the like, to facilitate mobility for those who are physically impaired. Another aspect of this law involved an affirmative action component, which assured persons with disabilities equal opportunities for employment if they were otherwise qualified.

As noted, until the passage of Public Law 94-142 (the Education for All Handicapped Children Act of 1975), students with special needs were frequently excluded from public school attendance (Turnbull & Turnbull, 1986; Simpson, 1996). It should also be noted that prior to Public Law 94-142, several states had passed their own special education laws. However, these state-specific laws pertained only to the states in which they were passed (Bauer & Shea, 1999). Public Law 94-142 is by far the most comprehensive legislation on behalf of children with disabilities (Alper et al., 1994). This law compels states to provide education for *all* students with disabilities. Some of the requirements of Public Law 94-142 are as follows:

- Procedures for referring children suspected of having a disability.
- A team comprised of personnel from varied disciplines to determine eligibility.
- Team development of an Individualized Education Program (IEP).
- Specialized instruction and placement in an educational setting appropriate to the child's needs.
- Procedures for parental notification and participation.
- Time limits on how rapidly the eligibility/referral process occurs.
- Periodic reassessment of the student's eligibility.
- Procedures for resolving disagreements/disputes. (Bradley et al., 1997, p. 24)

The core of this legislation provides for a free and appropriate public education for all children and youth with disabilities. Furthermore, special education and related services must also be provided at public expense.

Public Law 94-142 was amended and renamed in 1990 and then

again since that time, as Individuals with Disabilities Act (IDEA; Public Law 101-476). The IDEA strengthened Public Law 94-142 by adding two new categories: (1) autism and traumatic brain injury, and (2) added transition plans for 16-year-olds (now age 14) with disabilities. Instead of focusing only on academic objectives, these plans focused on life beyond school, including employment, education, residence, and leisure activities; and provided for services to individuals with disabilities from 0 to 21 years (F. Prezant, personal communication, June 15, 1999).

The most complex provision of Public Law 94-142 is the notion of what constitutes an appropriate education. Based on the law, yet open to interpretation and debate (Bauer & Shea, 1999), schools must provide individualized instruction based on an assessment of a child's needs. Furthermore, related services such as speech and physical therapy may be required to provide a comprehensive educational program. Both a multidisciplinary team and the parents are to be involved in the development of the IEP. A key element of the law is that educational programs must be provided in the least restrictive environment appropriate to the characteristics of the student. Related to the processes and decisions derived from the IEP conference, Public Law 94-142 includes families' rights to due process.

The Education of the Handicapped Act Amendments of 1986 extended Public Law 94-142 downward; that is, 5-year-old and younger children with disabilities were protected under the law, the same as children age five years and older under Public Law 94-142. The law, 99-457, provides children ages 3 to 21 with a right to a free and public education in Part B; and in Part H, this law provides incentives for working with infants and toddlers with disabilities. Instead of an IEP, the amendments require the use of an Individualized Family Service Plan (IFSP). IFSPs are generally conducted in early childhood intervention programs and provide for a comprehensive service delivery approach to both the child's and the family's needs (Seligman & Darling, 1997; Bauer & Shea, 1999). An IFSP contains the following:

(1) a statement of the infant's or toddler's present levels of physical, cognitive, language, speech, psychosocial development, and self-help skills is provided, based on acceptable objective criteria,

(2) a statement of the family's strengths and needs relating to enhancing the development of the family's infant or toddler with a disability,

(3) a statement of the major outcomes expected to be achieved for the infant or toddler and the family, and the criteria, procedures, and timelines used to determine the degree to which progress toward achieving the outcomes or services necessary,

(4) a statement of specific early intervention services necessary to meet the unique needs of the infant or toddler and the family, including the frequency, intensity, and the method of delivering services,

(5) the projected dates for initiation of services and the anticipated duration of such services,

(6) the name of the case manager from the profession most immediately relevant to the infant's or toddler's or family's needs who will be responsible for the implementation of the plan and coordination with other agencies and persons, and

(7) the steps to be taken supporting the transition of the toddler with a disability to service provided under subchapter II of this chapter to the extent such services are considered appropriate. (U.S.C., Section 1477(d)(1-7), in Bradley et al., 1997, p. 25)

IFSPs can be facilitated by the use of a Parent Needs Survey (PNS). A sample PNS adapted from Seligman and Darling (1997) is included in Figure 7.1, which is based on the research by Darling and Baxter (1996). According to the literature, there are six major areas of need or concern in this population:

1. *Information* about diagnosis, prognosis, and treatments.
2. *Intervention* for the child—medical, therapeutic, and educational.
3. *Formal support* from public and private agencies.
4. *Informal support* from relatives, friends, neighbors, coworkers, and other parents.
5. *Material support,* including financial support and access to resources.
6. Elimination of *competing family needs,* that is, needs of other family members (parents, siblings, etc.) that may affect the family's ability to attend to the needs of the child with a disability.

The Americans with Disabilities Act (ADA) of 1990 is directed to the needs of adults with disabilities. Children with disabilities eventually become adults and adult children with disabilities (Marshak et al., 1999). The chief goal of this act is to reduce segregation

FIGURE 7.1. Parent Needs Survey. Adapted from Seligman and Darling (1997). Copyright 1997 by The Guilford Press. Adapted by permission.

Date: _____

Name of person completing form: _____

Relationship to child: _____

Parents of young children have many different needs. Not all parents need the same kinds of help. For each of the needs listed below, please check (×) the space that best describes your need or desire for help in that area. Although we may not be able to help you with all your needs, your answers will help us improve our program.

	I really need some help in this area.	I would like some help, but my need is not that great.	I don't need any help in this area.
1. More information about my child's disability.			
2. Someone who can help me feel better about myself.			
3. Help with child care.			
4. More money/financial help.			
5. Someone who can babysit for a day or evening so I/we can get away.			
6. Better medical care for my child.			
7. More information about child development.			
8. More information about behavior problems.			
9. More information about programs that can help my child.			
10. Counseling to help me cope with my situation.			
11. Better/more frequent teaching or therapy services for my child.			
12. Day care so I can get a job.			
13. A bigger or better house or apartment			
14. More information about how I can help my child.			
15. More information about nutrition or feeding.			

(*continued on next page*)

FIGURE 7.1. (*continued*)

	I really need some help in this area.	I would like some help, but my need is not that great.	I don't need any help in this area.
16. Learning how to handle my other children's jealousy of their brother or sister.			
17. Problems with in-laws or other relatives.			
18. Problems with friends or neighbors.			
19. Special equipment to meet my child's needs.			
20. More friends who have a child like mine.			
21. Someone to talk to about my problems.			
22. Problems with my husband (wife).			
23. A car or other form of transportation.			
24. Medical care for myself.			
25. More time for myself.			
26. More time to be with my child.			

Please list any needs we have forgotten:

27.			
28.			
29.			
30.			
31.			
32.			
33.			
34.			

and discrimination of individuals, namely, to assure quality of opportunity, independent living, full participation, and economic self-sufficiency. The law requires that all reasonable accommodations be made for persons with disabilities in such areas as housing, transportation, recreation, and facilities. An important aspect of this legislation is that businesses with more than 14 employees cannot discriminate against individuals with disabilities in hiring, advancement, and during the application and discharge process. This legislation also authorizes transition services to promote movement from school to postschool activities.

As articulated by Turnbull and Turnbull (1986) these key legislative initiatives have led to the following six principles of special education law:

1. *Zero-reject*: Schools must educate all children with disabilities and may not exclude any school-age children solely because the child has a disability.
2. *Nondiscriminatory evaluation*: Schools must test and classify children fairly, essentially by administering non-biased tests in ways that do not put children at a disadvantage but that allow them to display their educational abilities and disabilities.
3. *Appropriate, individualized education*: Schools must provide each child with an individually tailored education.
4. *Least restrictive educational placement*: Schools must educate children who have disabilities with their peers who do not have disabilities to the greatest extent consistent with their educational and social needs.
5. *Procedural due process*: Schools must provide opportunities for children's parents to consent or object to their children's educational identification, classification, program, or placement.
6. *Parent participation*: Parents of children with disabilities may participate in various ways in their children's education. (p. 170)

WHAT CONSTITUTES THE IEP?

The IEP describes the educational and related services designed to meet the needs of children with disabilities (Anderson, Chitwood, & Hayden, 1997; Friend & Bursuck, 1999). A child's program is developed during the IEP meeting and specified in writing in an IEP planning document.

Written Components of an IEP Plan

Parents play a central role in the development of the planning document, which contains six components. Actually, the IEP is developed by parents, educators, and other relevant professionals, and sometimes in the presence of the child. The document specifies the educational placement (or setting) and the related services (e.g., speech therapy, transportation) needed to achieve the written objectives. It includes dates when services are initiated and terminated, and indicates how a child's progress is measured. According to Anderson et al. (1997), the IEP is a written commitment of the educational and adjunct services the school agrees to provide. Parents and school personnel agree on periodic reviews of the planning document, which provide for an assessment of the child's progress toward meeting the established goals. These are the six components of an IEP.

Description of the Child

The IEP written document must contain certain elements (Anderson et al., 1997; Turnbull & Turnbull, 1986; Lambie, 2000). The first ingredient is a description of the child, which include's such basic information as name, age, and so on. A child's current level of educational and behavioral performance is included, as well as how the disability effects achievement. Parents have a unique opportunity here to highlight their child's learning style, which could have a bearing on the educational methods employed.

Goals and Objectives

The second IEP ingredient is the establishment of goals and objectives designed to meet the child's needs. These goals and objectives are measured against the child's current level of functioning. Goals should be observable, measurable, and clearly describe the behavior in question. Anderson et al. (1997) provide examples of vague and well-constructed goal statements. Ambiguous goals are confusing and may lead to interpretation difficulties.

Vague goals
- Bonnie Jean will improve her self-concept.
- Edward will communicate better.
- Nina will be cooperative.

Well-constructed goals

- Edward will use sign language to ask for bathroom priviledges by June 30.
- Nina will prepare and present an oral report in social studies with two general education classmates by May 7.

Related Services

Ancillary services help augment and support the educational program for a child. These services, which are free to the parents, are designed to help children gain maximum benefit from their education in the least restrictive environment. Related services may include but are not limited to the following:

- Medical services
- Audiology
- Assistive technology
- Counseling
- Occupational and physical services
- Speech and language services
- Transportation

These adjunct services must be written into the IEP. Similar to the articulation of educational services and goals in the IEP, related services must also be clearly written with specific goals, activities, and time lines. Anderson et al. (1997, p. 86) provide examples of poorly and well-written statements:

> *Not acceptable*: "Bonnie Jean will receive speech therapy" or "Bonnie Jean will receive adaptive PE"
> *Acceptable*: "Bonnie Jean will speak in three-word sentences using noun, verb, and object in the classroom by May 15."

Once it is determined by the parents and the school that a child needs related services, the school system is legally obligated to provide them in the least restrictive environment, even when those services do not presently exist within the school system.

Special Education Placement

In the past, children with disabilities were placed in classrooms based on disability groupings (Anderson et al., 1997). For example, students with mental retardation, learning disabilities, and physical impairments were placed in classrooms with other students who had the same disability. Now, placement is derived from the goals and objectives included in the IEP and not based on disability type. The placement decision is made on the basis of a child's needs and strengths, and where the child's goals can be appropriately implemented and achieved. Placement decisions are ultimately made on the basis of an appropriate educational program and the least restrictive environment. According to Public Law 94-142:

> It is the purpose of this Act to assume that all children with disabilities have available to them . . . a free, appropriate, public education which emphasizes special education and related services designed to meet their unique needs. To the maximum extent appropriate, children with disabilities, including children in public or private institutions or other care facilities, are educated with children who are not disabled. (in Anderson et al., 1997, p. 46)

In 1982, the U.S. Supreme Court, clarified the term "appropriate education" by reinforcing the notion that an appropriate education is individualized to the needs of the child (Anderson et al., 1977). Furthermore, if a child does not progress as envisioned by the IEP team (parents and school personnel), the parents can question the placement and call for a special meeting of the IEP committee. An important aspect of placement concerns a focus on a child's ability, not just disability—both strengths and needs are taken into consideration.

Before an appropriate placement decision is reached, the parents and the educational team need to consider the least restrictive environment (LRE) in which a student can maximize academic and social learning. Those who determine a child's LRE should consider the extent to which he or she can be educated with nondisabled students. Bauer and Shea (1999) define LRE as "the environment in which learners with disabilities can succeed that is most similar to the environment in which his or her peers are educated" (p. 30). Segregated learning environments discourage the development of friendships between students with and without disabilities and limit their opportunities for learning from one another. Also, integrated settings may help ease the transition between schools and community living for many children with disabilities. The social dimension of a child's education is deemed to be important in that it can influence future vocational endeavors, friendships, community living, and family dynamics.

Anderson et al. (1997) note that a child's appropriate education and LRE should be given equal consideration. LRE does not necessarily mean that all children be placed into general education classrooms. Again, the appropriateness of the placement must be taken into consideration, along with an environment that is least restrictive.

Time and Duration of Services

The starting times and duration of a child's educational activities are determined. Furthermore, the school system has an obligation to begin services in a timely manner. A typical time-and-duration statement may be something like the following: "David will engage in physical therapy three times weekly for 1 hour. The service will begin on January 28, 2002, and end May 31, 2002."

Evaluating the IEP

Once an IEP planning document is written and implemented, it is imperative that parents and teachers schedule subsequent meetings designed to review a child's progress. The meeting is intended to review the goals and objectives established in the IEP. The precise nature of the written goals and time frame allows parents and teachers to discuss each activity and determine whether there has been positive movement. Review meetings should be scheduled at least yearly and at other times when parents or teachers ask for them.

The following is a hypothetical illustration of what can happen when schools fail to heed the purpose and intent of the law in preparing for and conducting an IEP conference (Marshak et al., 1999):

A child with learning disabilities, attention deficits, and a bipolar disorder is doing poorly in school. An evaluation is requested and assessment results indicate the child is functioning at low levels academically. The team fails to request parent input even thought the parent has demonstrated interest. The parent has no knowledge of due process rights to be involved. Limited testing is conducted in the area of achievement, with no assessments of the child's intellectual potential. Observations reveal a child who does not follow classroom directions, does not pay attention, and is frequently reprimanded by the teacher and excluded by classmates. The team decides that the child has some disciplinary problems due to lack of parental interest and that the child does not meet eligibility requirements for any specific category, but could use more discipline and attention at home.

A meeting is scheduled and for the first time the parents are invited to participate in the process. At the meeting, they are astonished to hear the findings and finally share information regarding outside help the child has been receiving. The team sticks by its decision. The parents consult with their mental health professionals and someone puts them in touch with a local parent advocacy group. When they find out about their rights, they ask for an independent evaluation, which the school denies. A prehearing conference ensues and then a hearing. It is then up to the school district to prove that its evaluation was appropriate. Upon finding that the parents' rights were violated, that they were not part of the process, and that the evaluation was incomplete, the hearing officer agrees that an independent evaluation is needed and the school district must pay the cost. The family has the child thoroughly evaluated by a neuropsychologist, incorporating reports from the psychiatric and other mental health professionals who have been serving the child. This comprehensive evaluation demonstrates that the child may meet the criteria for three categories (other health impairments, learning disability, and serious emotional disturbance) and that there is an indisputable need for specialized instruction. The fact that these professionals write that the child needs these services to make meaningful progress rather than saying only that the child might benefit from them is significant.

An IEP is written with input from the outside professionals whom the parents invite to the meeting. The IEP is implemented and the child receives language therapy, school-based counseling in conjunction with outside consultation, resource room assistance for two periods a day, and regular classroom placement for the rest of the day. It is decided that periodic reports will be forwarded to the outside professionals and to the parents to coordinate efforts.

Clearly, not all IEP's are developed under such adversarial conditions. Most run smoothly and schools in general do a good job of evaluating children and involving parents in the process. To ensure that everyone understands his or her role and impact, it is critical that all parties comprehend the rights, the rules, the process, and the purpose of the IEP. (pp. 120–121)

Due Process

In regard to parents' right to due process, Simpson (1996) writes, "Probably, no single phrase in education produces such a visceral response as due process. Both parents and educators alike seem to associate it with legal involvement, conflict, and proceedings more aligned with a courtroom than an educational setting" (p. 192). Essentially, due process hearings come about when either parents or the school disagree over recommendations made about a child's educational program.

Due process in education was initially presented in *Pennsylvania Association for Retarded Children v. Commonwealth of Pennsylvania,* in 1972 (Simpson, 1996), later to become the Education for All Handicapped Children Act, enacted by Congress in 1975. The basic ideas of due process articulated in 1972 are currently contained in the Individuals with Disabilities Act (IDEA). The IDEA was reauthorized in 1997, and contains greater expectations and opportunities for inclusion of children with special needs (Autin, 1999). The child's IEP must now include the general education classes that he or she attends. It must also articulate any necessary adaptations that must be made to accommodate inclusion. Children with special needs must be exposed to the services and programs available to nondisabled children, such as art, music, homemaking, physical education, and the like.

Due to the emphasis on inclusion, the 1997 reauthorization of the IDEA specifies that training and professional development opportunities for the general education teacher be provided. The purpose of the training is to increase the competence of general educators in teaching children with disabilities and in conferring with their parents. The training of general education teachers will also help to decrease the schism that has existed between general and special education (Autin, 1999; Marshak et al., 1999) that has led to conflict and jealousies between these educators, and a fragmented and disconnected practice of inclusion. It is expected that increased inclusion will be facilitated by more frequent and meaningful collaboration between general and special educators.

Due process procedures also give parents and children access to records, independent evaluations, surrogate parents, parental notice, and right to a hearing. Simpson (1996) addresses these elements: *Parental access to records* means that parents or legal guardians have access to records of their children. *Independent evaluations* mean that parents are entitled to secure an evaluation of their child at public expense from a qualified professional not affiliated with the school or agency when parents disagree with the evaluation results provided by the school district. *Appointment of surrogate parents* is considered when a child is a ward of the state or the parents are unknown or unavailable. *Right to parental notice* means that the school must notify parents in writing whenever there is a decision to evaluate a child or change an educational program. Parents are also required to notify the school in writing when they plan evaluations or changes. *Right to a hearing* allows parents and the school an opportunity for an objective hearing that ultimately leads to the most appropriate educational placement for a child.

Anderson et al. (1997) believe that a due process hearing should be the parents' last resort for achieving appropriate educational placement for their child. They argue that differences of opinion are best resolved in a more informal environment, starting with the teacher and, if needed, a meeting with the teacher and other school officials. Some schools provide opportunities to participate in mediation before resorting to a due process hearing. Mediation is often recommended for fighting martial partners before resorting to attorneys and endless court battles. Marital issues are intensified and prolonged when they reach the courts. Likewise, conflict and lingering negative emotions can be the legacy of a due process hearing.

As noted earlier, due process had its legislative birth in the Education for All Handicapped Children Act (1975) and was reauthorized as the IDEA (1990), which describes the procedures for due process hearings and identifies the conflicts that may be resolved by the process. Due process hearings are not intended to resolve all disputes.

Parents can *only* initiate a due process procedure when the school system has violated a duty it is required to perform by law (Anderson et al., 1997). Specifically, the IDEA requires the following:

1. School systems must provide a free, appropriate public education for all children with disabilities, age 3 through 21, unless state law prohibits or does not authorize the expenditure of public funds to educate children without disabilities, age 3 through 5 or 18 through 21.
2. School systems must ensure that children with and without disabilities are educated together to the maximum extent appropriate.
3. School systems must set forth in writing in the IEP the specially designed education and related services children will receive to meet their unique educational needs.
4. School systems must give reasonable written notice to parents before they evaluate or place a child, change special education placement, or refuse to take such actions.
5. School systems must obtain parental consent before the initial evaluation is conducted and before the child is first placed in a special education program on the basis of the IEP.

6. School systems must provide an evaluation of the child using a multidisciplinary team, which includes at least one teacher or other specialist knowledgeable in the area of the suspected disability.

7. School systems must ensure that evaluation tests are nondiscriminatory.

8. School systems must make available to parents for inspection and review all records used in the evaluation, placement, and IEP processes, as well as those records that are a part of the child's official school file.

9. School systems must provide for the child an *independent evaluation* at public expense if the parents disagree with evaluation results obtained by the school system.

10. Upon request, school systems must provide an impartial due process hearing to parents who believe any of the preceding rights have been violated.

Anderson et al. (1997) provide the following examples of the types of conflicts that are subject to resolution in due process hearings:

• Whether a child should be identified as having a learning disability or emotional disturbance (evaluation/eligibility).

• Whether a child should be placed in a self-contained classroom or a general education classroom with support services (LRE).

• Whether a child should be placed at public expense in a private school (appropriate education and LRE).

• Whether a specific intelligence test discriminates against young, nonverbal children (nondiscriminatory testing and the need for an independent evaluation).

• Whether a child is receiving the program outlined in her IEP or IFSP (appropriate education).

• Whether a child receives services at home or at a school (LRE).

It is useful at this juncture to reiterate the Anderson et al. (1997) caveat that a decision to pursue a due process hearing should take place only when parents believe that their rights, as stipulated here, have been violated. In this regard, these authors caution parents:

The decision to resolve your differences with the school system through due process hearing should not be taken lightly. These steps will ultimately involve significant time, money, thought, and physical and emotional energy from both you (the parent) and school people. Consequently, it is seldom advisable to seek a due process hearing unless you have reached the point where you feel any further discussions with school officials are futile and the only way around the impasse is a hearing. Before you reach this point, use every possible means to resolve disagreements. Attend meetings. Request conferences with the teacher, principal, or special education director. Listen to and seriously consider all proposed solutions. Ask questions. And provide all the information you have to prove that your view or recommendation is correct. Prior to requesting a hearing, you may wish to try an intermediate step. In your state this step may be called an administrative review, a conciliatory conference or mediation. (p. 176)

Due process procedures have promoted the intent of the IDEA in two ways (Anderson et al., 1997). First, the reality of due process puts schools on notice that their actions can be reviewed by an impartial process. Consequently, "school officials have become more careful, discreet, objective, and open in their work. Without the cloud of the due process hearing hanging over their heads, many school systems might lapse into the practices of prior years where parents' concerns were ignored or merely tolerated" (p. 181).

Second, because of the volume of students served by the schools each year, mistakes are made. Because of the IDEA, the IEP process, and due process hearings, mistakes need not go uncorrected. These procedures assure parents that their voice will be heard along with educators and others who comprise the professional team.

The Collaborative Effort

In addition to the focus on the educational program per se, the IEP has another, perhaps less discussed, *raison d'être*. Just as children are better served by an intact family or even divorced parents who communicate with each other, a child's educational plan becomes a truly useful document when both parents and teachers enjoy good relations and effectively collaborate. To this end, Turnbull and Turnbull, (1986) offer the following nuggets of good advice to teachers in their efforts to collaborate with parents:

Professionals who want to carry out the parent–professional opportunities of the IEP will do the following: (a) strive to have parents present; (b) inform parents that the student may be present and even suggest that the student should be present; (c) respect parents' opinions about the student's abilities and disabilities; (d) be particularly careful to respect parents' opinions about what program the student should have, because, in most cases and in the final analysis, parents (not professionals) are the people ultimately responsible for their children; (e) avoid using educational jargon and be clear in communicating with parents, especially in communicating why they believe the student should be placed in a certain program and why the objectives and evaluation methods in the proposed IEP are proposed; (f) look on the IEP meeting as an opportunity to work with each other and with parents to obtain shared decision making, shared accountability for the student's program, and shared commitment to appropriate education. (p. 182)

Most professionals recognize that families come in many forms and are indeed dynamic and complex systems (Lambie, 2000; Bauer & Shea, 1999). Personal values and opinions can also contribute to the usual complexities of family life. Generally speaking, family members have a variety of opinions on any number of topics. Therefore, there are value and opinion differences that make for spicy dinnertime conversations. Some differences are expected and should be explored and respected; other differences lead to arguments, confrontations, and even major conflict.

During conferences, a teacher needs to be sensitive to parents who may wish to have their child in a segregated setting when she believes their child can do well in an inclusive setting. She can give her opinion but, as the Turnbull's suggested earlier, the teacher must respect the parents' decision. By providing cogent reasons for inclusion, the teacher may be able to dissuade parents from a decision that they believe is not ideal for their child, but again, the teacher should be sensitive to the parents' wishes and perhaps even endeavor to understand what might be behind their choice, especially if she believes their decision is ill advised.

A challenging situation can arise when parents disagree with each other over placement or the least restrictive involvement. Under these circumstances, there may be an impasse borne of legitimate differences of opinion. On the other hand, strong opinions can reflect underlying family conflict. For example, a teacher might witness an emotional confrontation between parents on the subject of what is in the child's best interest. On the surface, the argument appears to reflect a true difference of opinion. Upon further observation and reflection, the teacher can see that the parents do not agree on any issues that emerge during the conference. This dynamic can suggest a power struggle or control issues that have been brought into the parent–teacher meeting.

It can be difficult to discern whether you are observing a power struggle or an honest disagreement between the parents on a crucial educational decision. You can generally tell as the conference continues, and the parents either continue in a tension-filled manner or in a more congenial discussion of the issue. Certainly, because the issue is so important, parents may argue with some emotion over their child's educational future, without an indication of marital problems. However, if it is certain that what is transpiring during the conference is the reflection of a more general problem, you can listen for a while, then attempt to redirect the session to refocus the interaction. For example:

"From the discussion so far I can see that you are both concerned about your child's educational placement. I am pleased to see that you have your child's interest at heart. But, I wonder whether you might find it more helpful to discuss this important issue at length at home, where you can discuss the merits of an inclusive versus segregated setting. After you have reached a decision, please call me and we can begin to discuss the implementation of the decision. In the meantime, I wonder if we can get back to the issue of _____."

A more controversial course of action would be to state that you sense an underlying conflict that is being expressed through the admittedly difficult educational decision about their child. I would argue against this approach, because you are the child's teacher, not the parents' therapist. Also, once the issue is laid bare, it is possible that parents would thrust you into the role of arbiter or therapist and expect you to help them resolve their underlying conflicts. On the other hand, they may resent a teacher's intrusion into their personal lives.

As we know from the discussion thus far, the IEP meeting involves more than just the parents and the teacher. It generally includes a team of professionals involved in a child's education and welfare, from teachers to speech and physical therapists, and the like. As already discussed, meeting with a team of professionals can be intimidating for parents. According to Simpson (1996), many parents report experiencing anxiety at these meetings. Others feel they are not prepared to contribute in a helpful manner.

To help reduce the intimidation factor, Simpson (1996) advises:

- No more participants than necessary should be allowed in the meeting. Although no one should be denied admission whose contribution may be of benefit, neither should the effective composition of the group be compromised by marginally involved persons. Indeed, Department of Education guidelines note that:

  The number of participants at IEP meetings should be small. Small meetings have several advantages over large ones. . . . They allow for more open, active parent involvement, are less costly, are easier to arrange and conduct, and are usually more productive. (Federal Register, 57[208], p. 48699)

- Nonessential and nonproductive "professionalism" should be eliminated from the session. In particular, an informal and friendly conference style can most effectively create an atmosphere of warmth for parents and a willingness to form partnerships.

- Parents should be encouraged to bring a friend or confidant to the conference, particularly someone who is familiar with the IEP process.

- Parents should have at least one professional at the conference with whom they are familiar and to whom they can relate. It is simply unrealistic to assume that parents can enter a group of professional strangers, without the benefit of at least one previously established relationship, and function as a contributing and collaborative member of an IEP team. (p. 217)

Because of the intimidating nature of an IEP, some have argued in favor of preparatory training for parents so that they will be better informed about the process and, consequently, feel more at ease (F. Prezant, personal communication, May 24, 1999). Indeed, Simpson (1996) believes that parents are at a distinct disadvantage during these meetings without training. Simpson and Fiedler (1989) recommend systematic training for parents and professionals so that both are prepared to have a successful IEP conference.

Impediments to Parents Participation

The reciprocal views of parents and teachers were addressed in Chapter 2. From that discussion it is clear that there are often misperceptions between parents and teachers that may fuel strained relationships between the two. This might be a good place to discuss and review these participants' contributions to a conference.

Turnbull and Turnbull (1986) note that there can be barriers to parents' participation. These authors believe that logistical and communication problems, and inadequate knowledge by parents reflect key areas of concern. Logistical problems might include lack of transportation, child care, and sufficient time during conferences; communication problems might include language and cultural differences; a lack of knowledge can contribute to parents' feelings of inferiority, uncertainty about a child's disability, and misunderstanding of how schools can help.

Logistical problems can be remedied in some unique situations by having conferences in community centers, churches, or synagogues. Meeting in parents' home can help alleviate child-care problems. Another major logistical problem is the inclusion of fathers in conferences. It is important to make every effort to arrange times so that fathers can attend. Meeting times need to be flexible, offering early morning, late afternoon, and evening or lunch hours (Turnbull & Turnbull, 1986). The school administration needs to approve of flexible hours so that teachers feel supported in having them.

Communication problems chiefly occur around language and cultural barriers. To help minimize communication problems, teachers can work with churches and other organizations within minority communities. Having a translator, if needed, summarizing the decisions made during meetings, not using professional jargon, and providing a concise written summary of the meeting's key points can reduce communication difficulties. Translators may be included only after receiving the parents' permission. The material discussed during conferences can be highly personal; therefore, the selection of a translator should be endorsed by the parents.

School personnel must be careful to not coerce parents into any action by taking advantage of language and cultural differences (Harry, 1992). Parents from other cultures may not ask important questions relating to their child's educational program, or by virtue of cultural sanctions that one does not question those in authority, they may not be willing to challenge decisions. Harry points out how parents from other cultures may be physically present at an IEP conference yet be essentially locked out of any meaningful participation:

> Although parents are invited to be present and participate, there is no escaping the fact that they are respondents in the situation. Indeed, the data of this study show unequivocally that culturally different parents come to these meetings as strangers to a system that is legally required to include them, but whose patterns of discourse are so structured as

to exclude meaningful dialogue, and, indeed, to delegitimate parents' views. . . . While parents' own personal styles will have an impact on the proceedings, it is essentially the structure and atmosphere provided that will either include or exclude parents. (p. 230)

Mainstream and minority parents may lack information about their legal rights. As reported earlier, key figures in the field urge parents to participate in preconference training workshops (Simpson, 1996; Turnbull & Turnbull, 1986; Harry, 1992). Research indicates that parents fare better in IEP meetings after some type of preconference education (Thompson, 1982; Malmberg, 1984). Parents can be prepared through simulated activities, audiovisual tapes, discussion, or written materials. By engaging in preparatory activities, parents may feel more appropriately assertive and satisfied with the conference experience.

Feelings of inferiority during meetings may stem from experiencing reduced status in decision making, feelings of intimidation, as noted earlier, because of being outnumbered by professionals at IEP meetings, and perhaps also because of a lingering doubt that they may be the cause of the child's disability. To help parents feel more comfortable during meetings, the teacher can treat them as valued members of the decision-making team (Pistono, 1977). Rather than being treated as passive participants, parents should be regarded as partners with deep concerns about their child's educational future.

Sometimes the significant differences in education and social class between parents and professionals can be another intimidating factor. Parents may feel uneasy in the presence of highly educated professionals who have specific specialties. Ultimately, the reduction of parental anxiety is best achieved when professionals are respectful of the parenting role and treat parents with kindness, empathy, and support.

Parents with children whose disabilities are milder or without a known etiology can be uncertain about the child's exceptionality (Fewell, 1991; Seligman & Darling, 1997). This type of situation may be more challenging for professionals and parents to address at an IEP conference. For the professional, this is not a place to "show off" diagnostic skills; a misdiagnosis can result in agony for the parents. If appropriate, professionals can hypothesize *along with the parents* on how certain behaviors or symptoms *may* relate to a particular condition. Here, again, teachers need to be well informed about their role.

According to studies, parents are not typically perceived as making significant contributions to IEP meetings, perhaps because of the reasons just cited (Gilliam & Coleman, 1981). This finding is somewhat perplexing in that parents are deeply concerned about their child's academic and emotional well-being, yet perhaps as a consequence of the anxiety-provoking nature of the IEP conference, they may fail to assert themselves on behalf of their children. Intimidation is a factor in parental reluctance to participate actively, but some educators argue that parents may not know how to participate effectively (Harry, 1992).

Again, cultural differences, may interfere with participation. One study found that the frequency of parental suggestions during IEPs was influenced by cultural factors; for example, Latino parents offered fewer suggestions than African American or Caucasian parents (Lynch & Stein, 1982). In response, then, it is incumbent upon teachers to reduce parental anxiety and facilitate parental preparation and participation in the IEP and other meetings.

Before an IEP meeting, parents may wish to talk with their child to determine whether he or she wishes to attend the meeting (Gillespie & Turnbull, 1983). Questions parents may wish to keep in mind as they consider having their child attend include whether the child will understand the language used in the conference and be able to communicate specific preferences and wishes. Some consideration should be made in regard to a child's comfort given the possibility of disagreement and tension during the meeting. However, the value of having children present is so that they can experience some control over their lives and not feel that the meetings are secretive discussions about them, and, like other family events, so they can feel included.

Other Elements of Parent–Teacher Meetings

The barometer of any successful interpersonal encounter is the degree to which the participants can achieve rapport. When rapport is absent, there are more disagreements, conflict, tension, and chances for a poor outcome.

Rapport is easily ruptured when professionals are insensitive, even when these actions are not intentional (Beckman, 1996), for example, when no one introduces the parents to the professionals at a conference, or when someone talks about a family member as if she were not present. Referring to parents as "mom" or "dad" helps to define the relationship between the professionals and parents as unequal (Leviton, Muellen, & Kauffmann, 1992).

Sometimes, without being aware of what they are doing, professionals may overemphasize a child's negative aspects, while ignoring the positive ones. One mother expressed her dismay thusly: "Even when I get all the services I want for my son, I never fail to leave the meetings with a lump in my throat. It is still so hard to hear about all of the things he *can't* do that other children his age can do" (in Beckman, 1996, p. 95).

Blaming parents for their child's disability is another concern. A couple of studies affirm that a major factor related to dissatisfaction with conferences is the extent to which parents are blamed by school officials for their child's problems (Witt, Miller, McIntyre, & Smith, 1984; Petr & Barney, 1993). Therefore, teachers and other school professionals need to be alert to inadvertently making observations that can be construed as blaming.

Another source of concern for parents is the time constraints of conferences (Beckman, 1996; Harry, 1992). To attend a meeting when there is insufficient time for questions or concerns is frustrating for parents. In addition, it is rude for team members to leave before the meeting is over because of "other commitments." Professionals attending parent conferences should abide by the same time frame that was initially decided. However, a professional who has interacted with the parents to their satisfaction, and whose presence is no longer needed, may exit with a few positive comments, such as "I apologize, but I must excuse myself from the meeting. I trust that I have been responsive to all of your questions. If you have any other questions or observations, I would welcome a call from you. In the meantime, you are in good hands with us. We will work with you to achieve an appropriate educational outcome for Tim. It was a pleasure meeting you."

It is prudent to schedule enough time for both parents and professionals to attend to all of the issues that need to be addressed. However, unstructured, open-ended, endless meetings can also be counterproductive. All of the parties present at a conference (including the parents) have other obligations and responsibilities. Comprehensive yet goal-oriented and comfortably paced meetings should be the goal. I believe that if parents have a few nonessential questions after a meeting, the teacher can, if time permits, field a few more queries. Such a simple act of kindness and concern on the part of the teacher can go a long way toward ensuring parents' overall satisfaction with the meeting, as can inviting the parents' phone call to tie up loose ends.

Teachers can make IEPs and other parent meetings less stressful and more productive by paying attention to some conference-related dynamics (Beckman & Stepanek, 1996). As other authors have noted, both strengths and areas of concern should be honestly communicated with kindness and support rather than in a manner that is harsh, rushed, or punishing. Note the difference between these two comments made by a professional:

> "According to the test results, your son's IQ falls within the severe range. This means that there are a host of things that he will not be able to do or accomplish in his lifetime. The reality is that he will need a lot of services to help him stay at his present level of functioning."

> "David tests out at a range that suggests that he will need help with language development, reading, and certain practical skills. David will have access to teachers and other professionals who have worked with these challenges before and have helped other children make gains in areas where they needed help. It's clear to me that David has some good interpersonal skills, which will help him make friendships in school and boost his confidence. David may be faced with some challenges in his life, but he will also know accomplishments."

What about Teachers?

Much of the discussion in this chapter addressed issues related to the parents' experience of comfortable, productive parent–teacher meetings. With the exception of the section on teacher burnout in Chapter 8, little is said about the stresses and anxieties that teachers experience when they are expected to teach children, confer with parents, prepare IEP documents, or attend a due process hearing. Teaching can be a challenging endeavor in itself, but so can conferencing. What makes conferencing difficult is the lack of training in how better to understand families of children with disabilities and how to conduct an effective conference. This training deficiency is compounded by parents who challenge teachers' expertise during conferences. Most parents want the best for their children and make sincere efforts to work cooperatively with teachers to construct a viable educational plan. A minority of parents, however, can be rude, pushy, uncooperative, angry, and challenging. They present with difficult behaviors because they believe that this is the best way to relate to others. Perhaps some parents relate more aggressively because it is what they were taught by their parents. Others may believe that other people are not trustworthy, or they are expressing their need to control. Still other parents can be challenges for the teacher because they are anxious about their child's future and perhaps have not come to grips with parenting a child with a disability. Nonetheless, for a teacher, a conference with a pushy, angry parent can make for an unforgettable day.

A key element in helping teachers cope with the stress in their professional lives is administrative support (see Chapter 1). School principals and other administrators should be clear and reasonable in their demands of teachers. Communication is enhanced when school administrators keep teachers informed about new legislation that affects education and any changes that are about to take place in the teacher's school. Administrators can communicate their support for their teachers' efforts and the national policy of inclusion. They can promote an open-door policy so that teachers can discuss issues as they arise or vent frustrations without retribution. Administrators can hold and/or encourage teacher meetings to discuss problems and issues that occur. Furthermore, administrators can allow teachers to attend conferences and workshops, where they can increase their teaching and conferencing skills. Just as teachers need to learn good interpersonal skills to effectively conduct parent–teacher meetings, so must administrators learn good communicating skills, so that teachers perceive them as allies and not adversaries.

In addition to conferences that increase skills and enhance self-confidence, teachers can utilize stress reduction exercises to help them remain calm during or after a conference. There are numerous books (e.g., McKay & Fanning, 1997; Bourne, 1990) on stress reduction, and many mental health professionals offer stress reduction workshops. Stress is a universal phenomenon in the speedy, impatient world in which we live. In fact, chronic stress has been confirmed to be a contributor to medical illness and to such psychological reactions as anxiety and depression.

Most of all, there needs to be recognition of teachers' expanded roles. Teaching and conferencing are both rewarding and stressful activities. A teacher's constitution and manner of coping determine how stressful teaching and conferencing can become. With administrative support, opportunities to discuss issues, and stress-reducing activities, teachers should be able to experience the pleasures of teaching children and conferencing with parents.

This chapter has explored the legislation that forms the cornerstone of the rights that children with disabilities and their families now enjoy after years of struggle to be included in the educational mainstream, and the two key mechanisms to emerge from legislative initiatives, namely, the IEP document and meeting, and the due process hearing. Impediments to successful IEP meetings were discussed along with parental anxieties about these conferences. Finally, the additional roles and expertise expected of teachers was discussed along with the concomitant stresses teachers face.

The final chapter focuses on parental personalities and behaviors that pose challenges to teachers during parent–teacher conferences.

8

Working with
Challenging Parents

As noted in Chapter 2, the general conclusion appears to be that teachers view parents more negatively than parents perceive teachers. Parents who behave in certain ways or possess certain attributes are considered to be "problem parents" and, as a result, challenge the teacher's interpersonal skills. It is helpful to understand that parents who are experienced as challenges may become problematic because of the teacher's reaction to them, or because the interaction between the parties is conflicted. However, the parent who is a problem for one teacher might not be for another. Due to personality characteristics and interpersonal style, teacher a meeting with parent a might be much more compatible than if parent a met with teacher b, whose characteristics would clash with those of the parent. Therefore, for some, the designation "problem parent" is misleading. What may be reflected in a problem situation are differences attributable to the interaction, not to either parent or teacher.

Sometimes teachers perceive parents accurately, as they really are; other times, parents are viewed by teachers in a distorted way, perhaps because of cultural stereotypes and/or personal anxiety. It is probably true that the dynamics of most parent–teacher encounters are a combination of reality and distortion on the part of both participants. It is important to be aware of the causal factors that influence perceptions, because only through such understanding will teachers be in a better position to appraise parents' behavior accurately.

I wrote the following discussion with some trepidation. Parents of children with disabilities have been categorized and characterized in a most unfavorable light, especially in the early literature; this situation creates negative attitudes toward them and feeds stereotypes (Seligman & Seligman, 1980; Sonnenschein, 1980). In addition, there is danger of generalizing when singling out "troublesome" characteristics of any particular group of people. It is important to keep in mind that the challenging parents examined in this chapter constitute a small minority of the parents that present themselves to teachers.

HOSTILE PARENTS

The apparent source of a parent's angry feelings may be the teacher, the school, or the curriculum. Anger might, of course, be directed toward institutions or people unrelated to the school the child attends (e.g., a physician or social worker). It is sometimes difficult to determine whether a parent's angry behavior and remarks can be taken at face value or whether they are manifestations of unconscious feelings related to factors unknown even to the parent. Knowledge of family dynamics and the common coping mechanisms described in Chapter 3 can help the teacher make more realistic appraisals of the causes of anger.

Perhaps the most anxiety-provoking, angry parent is the one who openly criticizes the teacher. The teacher may be accused of failing to cope with, teach, or in some other way meet the needs of the child. Criticism may be expressed in a rational, articulate fashion or with considerable emotion and animation. Although the teacher may perceive the anger as an attack on her person, in most cases, anger is projected; what appear to be angry feelings toward the teacher are really feelings that have been deflected from the original cause (e. g., anger over being a parent of a child with a disability) to the teacher. There are, of course, instances when parents' anger is justified.

Angry feelings directed at the school or teacher may indicate anxiety over the apparent lack of progress the child has made—through no fault of the teacher. It is sometimes easier to project blame onto another source than to face the reality of the disability. Some parents may be angry before they even meet their child's teacher because of past negative experiences with other professionals. Parents may legitimately be angered at the school for its inflexible policies or because they feel that their needs are neglected. Direct expressions of anger may also be indicative of the teacher's seeming lack of interest in them or their child. Some parents may be frustrated, feeling that the teacher places little value on their observations.

A particularly sensitive area, and a source of parental hostility, is when parents are told that their child will be transferred to another classroom or school. Such moves—where their child will be exposed to a new teacher, new peers, and a different environment—lead to considerable anxiety because the new situation involves a host of unknowns.

The teacher must be cognizant of veiled or indirect expressions of anger toward himself, the school, or the program in which the child is involved. The unexpressed portion of a parent's feelings about his child's general lack of progress may relate to perceived dissatisfaction with the teacher. However, such underlying feelings are difficult to uncover, and it is generally best not to assume blame or interpret the parent's comments as an indication of dissatisfaction with the teacher or school until the parent expresses it directly. In other words, the teacher may incorrectly say, "I think your unhappiness with Jim's progress suggests your dissatisfaction with me." A statement that would allow the parent a more open-ended response is "I sense your dissatisfaction with Jim's progress. Do you have any thoughts about why this is the case?" (For a discussion of the value of open-ended questions, see Chapter 6.)

In such instances, the teacher can relieve parental anger and impatience by indicating areas in which the child is making gains. Sometimes, in their impatience to see dramatic achievements, parents do not recognize the smaller gains their child has made.

The key to working with an angry parent is to avoid responding in a hostile or defensive way. Such responses contribute to a spiraling negative encounter in which both parties accuse each other of negligence and neither person listens to the other. Recall that the skill of listening is a powerful and positive response (Nichols, 1995), especially to people who are angry and feel that no one wants to hear their perspective.

With an uncharacteristically angry parent, a useful response would be a paraphrase and an open invitation to the parent to convey her perceptions:

> "Mrs. Cunningham, I can certainly understand your feelings of frustration and anger. You seem to be concerned about your daughter's behavior, which seems to have gotten worse since she has been in school. I wonder if you have any thoughts about why her behavior has changed?"

After listening to the parent, the teacher might wish to contribute her observations in an objective, noncontentious way. There will be times when the observations of parent and teacher coincide, as well as instances when they do not resemble each other at all. It is helpful to view differing perceptions in terms of complementary rather than contradictory observations. Observations by both parties are cumulative, adding to a more comprehensive picture of a situation.

The most productive reaction to angry expressions directed at sources outside of the school is to genuinely listen and then to paraphrase. For example, parents might be furious about an incident that painfully highlights their child's exceptionality. The angry feelings in such instances reflect both anger and hurt. In addition to attentive listening and paraphrasing, the teacher might wish to contribute supportive comments, such as, "It must have been painful to overhear a stranger make that thoughtless remark about David. However, it must be comforting for you to know that David's speech is intelligible to you and the rest of the family."

Critical, hostile parents are sometimes disarmed by a teacher who, rather than responding in kind, reacts in a nondefensive way. At other times, chronically hostile parents respond to a teacher who takes a firm and assertive stance (see Chapter 5). There is no easy way to learn assertive responses except through practice and self-monitoring. The growth of assertiveness training indicates the difficulty overly passive or exceedingly hostile people have in expressing their feelings in this manner. (The reader should have several opportunities to practice such responses through role-playing exercises in Chapter 6.)

Angry parents threaten the teacher more than any others. Indeed, most of us tend to avoid conflictual situations. More often than not, the anger reflects annoyance, frustration, or impatience at someone or something other than the teacher. By keeping this in mind, teachers will be less likely to personalize parental anger. By the same token, they must consider the possible validity of parents' observations, and when they have inadvertently erred, admission of the error reflects maturity and tends to enhance rapport.

UNCOOPERATIVE PARENTS

In addition to children who find various means to convey their lack of interest and cooperation in the classroom, parents likewise, by their uncooperative behavior, may be the source of considerable frustration for teachers who genuinely wish to form an alliance with them. It is useful to understand the reasons why parents may be uncooperative.

In some instances, parents may simply not have the time and energy to care. They may be preoccupied with family or work-related problems, or other problems of living. In other instances, they do care, but because of overwhelming burdens, they are, in fact, doing all they can to keep their lives together.

Anxiety can account for absences at parental conferences; hearing about a child's deficiencies is a painful reminder of a child's disability. Also, parents may agree to carry out a home program but find it difficult to implement. Avoidance (or withdrawal) may be the parents' way to keep anxiety at a manageable level.

The teacher may be faced with emotionally challenged or otherwise impaired parents whose involvement may be minimal. Invitations to come to conferences should be offered on occasion, but not in a threatening way. An invitation may be something like the following:

> "Although I realize that you are both struggling with some personal issues that we discussed previously on the phone, I, nevertheless, want to leave you with an open invitation to come in to discuss Peter's schooling. Feel free to call me, and if I am not available, leave a message and I will return your call."

Avoidance behavior may indicate that the parents are still denying or having difficulty coming to terms with their child's disability. During this period, the teacher ought to approach the parents cautiously, by realistically pointing out some areas where the child requires special help and others where she demonstrates strengths. When the teacher suspects parental denial, a greater focus on what the child does well rather than what she does poorly is recommended, yet one must be mindful that unrealistic statements about a child can deepen parental denial. Timing is especially critical here. The teacher wants to attract and welcome parents, not frighten them, and to remain realistic yet optimistic. It is not the teacher's duty to thrust painful reality upon a parent in the interest of developing parent–teacher cooperation. There are times when parents are open to feedback, but at other times, they may not be receptive. It is useful to recognize that one parent may be open to discussing the child, while the other is firmly in denial. One can observe this behavior during conferences, but I believe it is inappropriate for the teacher to attempt to thrust reality on parents when they are not prepared to accept it. Also, denial tends to fade to acceptance over time. It is helpful to keep in mind that parents experience different rates of movement from denial to a more realistic view of their child.

Some parents may feel that conferences are a formality, a school ritual of little substance. Others may be concerned that because of their modest education, they will not be looked upon favorably by the teacher or will be unable to understand what he says. Still others, because of faulty mail deliveries or frequent moves, are simply not notified of parent conferences.

Teachers must be wary of developing negative attitudes toward parents who miss conferences, sometimes without calling to cancel. To try to understand why conferences are missed, the teacher should gently and occasionally inquire, being careful not to imply wrongdoing. Here is an example: [On the phone] "Good to talk with you today about setting up another conference meeting. When you didn't show up last Tuesday at our scheduled meeting, I was worried that something may have happened. Is everything OK with both of you?"

Lack of cooperation may be a barometer of the relationship between parent and teacher, as most of us tend to avoid unpleasant interpersonal situations. Should the teacher be unable to ascertain the source of an impasse, an inquiry about the relationship is in order, such as, "You both seem to be less talkative over the past few conferences. Is there something that has occurred in our previous meetings that we need to discuss?"

At times, parents feel or perceive that teachers consider them to be a burden and, as a consequence, avoid contact with school personnel. They do not feel welcome and therefore are reluctant to collaborate with the teacher, even in the interest of their own child. The teacher should examine her own attitudes toward parents to determine whether there may be some negative attitudes that may carry over to the conference setting. When parents misconstrue the teacher's attitudes and she is aware of it, the teacher should undertake special efforts to make

the parents feel welcome. They can be encouraged to attend conferences, to help out in circumscribed ways in the classroom or with special activities and field trips, or be invited to observe their child in
school.

Some parents are so preoccupied with demanding jobs and/or
community activities that involvement in school would exceed their
available time and energy. However, being overly engaged with other
activities may be an excuse not to become involved with the child. This
coping mechanism needs to be understood, not challenged, as the
teacher should understand that anxious feelings about their child can
lead parents to engage in activities that lessen anxiety. Some parents
work tirelessly on behalf of disability causes, perhaps to avoid activities related to their own child. Other parents, who give of themselves
on the job and in the community, provide a caring environment for
their child at home but, because of their marginal involvement with
the teacher, appear to be disinterested and uncooperative. The teacher
should try to get to know these parents on the rare occasions that they
do meet, but she should not pressure them for more frequent conferences if they are disinclined to attend.

A teacher may wish to consider writing a note to the parent. Notes
should convey interest in meeting with the parent and a concern for
the child, not a veiled threat or a scolding. Occasional phone calls are
another available resource. Parents who are unable or do not wish to
attend conferences in person may be willing to talk to the teacher over
the phone. For some parents, phone conferences may be a stepping-
stone for future in-person meetings.

As an overriding rule, teachers should keep in mind that parents
will more willingly attend meetings when they know they will be conferring with a teacher who is knowledgeable, who listens, who seems
to like their child, and who cares. There is no easy solution for the resistance some parents demonstrate, however, and the teacher must be
alert to a developing apathy and resignation that may follow repeated
attempts to gain their cooperation. One can only benefit the child by
trying again.

PERFECTIONIST PARENTS (OR EXCESSIVELY WORRIED PARENTS)

In contrast to parents who eschew involvement with the school,
perfectionistic parents may be overly involved, particularly with their

child. For some, perfectionism can be traced to childhood, when achievements that were less than perfect were subject to criticism or ridicule. Even if the parents recognize at some level the deleterious effect their behavior has, the compulsion to demand perfection from others as well as themselves remains.

Perfectionistic parents express dismay to the child and the teacher when tasks are accomplished in a less than acceptable (usually perfect) fashion. The consequences of this type of behavior can be pronounced, as the child may be driven to achieve beyond his capabilities. Also, a child with a disability can be enormously frustrating to the perfectionist. Excessive parental tendencies of this kind can result in emotional problems for the child that complicate existing impediments. Almost certainly, the child will begin to develop a negative attitude toward schoolwork because of the barrage of criticism he receives whenever his performance falls below his parents' standard. The child's self-esteem suffers, further blocking whatever potential he may possess.

During conferences, it would be a mistake for the teacher to work toward a relaxation of the parents' unrealistically high standard. They should be made aware, however, in clear and understandable terms, the nature of the child's learning problems, his limitations, and his potential. An examination of the situations where the child functions optimally and those in which he does not should encourage the parents to realize that their child's progress is related both to psychological and cognitive factors. For example, without putting the parents on the defensive, the teacher might mention that when the child senses pressure in the classroom, his performance drops off considerably; conversely, when pressure is minimized, his performance generally improves. The teacher might try to explain that children respond differently to pressure; some thrive on it and others, finding it unbearable, react in an adverse way. Finally, the teacher might mention that praise and support when the child does well is a potent source of motivation. The parents might even be invited to observe their child in the classroom, but only if the teacher has some assurance that their presence will not have an adverse effect on the child, or vice versa.

If the teacher senses that only one of the parents is a perfectionist, she should try to encourage both parents to attend conferences. Of course, this is a good practice to follow in any event, but in such instances, the more rational parent can have a positive, counterbalancing effect on the perfectionist spouse.

It is important for the teacher to avoid indicating that the parent is at fault for the child's performance. The parent may already be aware of this and will gain further self-insight as the child performs better under less demanding circumstances.

PROFESSIONAL PARENTS

Some professional parents may be as threatening to a teacher as the teacher is to some parents. Much of the problem lies with the teacher's sense of awe; there are professional parents who consciously or unconsciously use their knowledge in a controlling or condescending way or, because of their position, demand special attention or favors for their child.

Professional parents may be more likely to get their way because school personnel want to please them for social and/or political reasons, or because they are more sophisticated at manipulating the system than those with less education and political savvy. One can hardly blame parents for wanting the best for their children, yet excessive and unrealistic demands should not be tolerated.

Professional parents who seem to annoy teachers most are those who feel that their knowledge about school, teaching, or educating children with disabilities gives them license to be unduly critical of the teacher or the curriculum. These parents may be motivated by their excessive concern for their child or their unconscious wish to impress the teacher with their knowledge, or simply by their need to exert influence and be in control. Parents who are frustrated teachers and somewhat knowledgeable but without credentials may also fall into this category. When receiving unsolicited advice from professional parents, as well as other parents, the teacher should weigh the advice to determine its merit and not automatically cast it aside. When a parent has a need to pass on her knowledge but does so in a sensible way, the teacher may wish to consider involving her in the classroom, but only if the teacher believes that the parent can function collaboratively.

Parents who are knowledgeable, as well as those who think they are, and attempt to interfere with the teaching program, the curriculum, or methods of discipline, require a different approach than interested parents who form helpful alliances with the teacher. Some interfering parents are appeased when given some small responsibilities to carry out; others become worse.

Scolding or arguing with parents yields little, but the teacher may need to set firm limits on what the parents do in the classroom. In terms of the conference, the teacher also has a right to assert her perception that the conference is to be used for making plans to help the child and not as a forum for constant criticism of the educational program. Although the parents' observations are welcome, the central focus of the conference is the child.

The advantage in this approach (of setting limits) is that the parent respects the professional expertise and integrity of the teacher. Also, the parent may covertly welcome the limits because they allow him to relax his need to demonstrate, whenever possible, his genuine concern and involvement for his child, or his feeling that the best way to demonstrate his knowledge is to exhibit it to the teacher whenever possible.

The potential risk of this response is to make the parent feel like a fool, a busybody, who has no right to convey his observations. The parent may complain to the principal or withdraw from the school altogether. In either case, the teacher should try to continue the dialogue so that feelings and perceptions of both parties become clear. Assertive behavior and limit setting should be considered when other possibilities have failed.

For the most part, professional parents are not substantially different from other involved parents. They tend to be concerned about their children, value education, promote a cooperative attitude, and, in general, are good team members. The disparity in status perceived by the teacher tends to be more of a problem than the actual behavior of a parent. In such circumstances, the teacher should remember that she is a trained specialist in teaching children, whereas the parent may be a specialist in another field. Information about their child, support, and encouragement are as important for these parents as they are for others.

DEPENDENT PARENTS

Dependent parents characteristically ask questions about virtually every aspect of the child's life. The dependent parent finds it difficult to assume the responsibility of making decisions; therefore, she enlists the help of the teacher in both minor and major matters. Because of a basic insecurity, the parent will solicit the teacher's opinions instead of risking her own.

A dependent parent generally cooperates with the teacher, although only when the teacher, not the parent, assumes responsibility for decisions and courses of action. A teacher who is working with a dependent parent sometimes wonders whether she is dealing with a child or an adult; overly dependent people do, in fact, resemble young children who cling to parents for direction and guidance. Perhaps the parent was never given responsibility as a child, or even after marriage, the spouse who was attracted to a dependent person may have further reinforced this behavior. Thus, the dependent parent rarely takes the opportunity to engage in independent thinking and subsequent responsibility.

Perhaps the parent feels that important decisions she made in the past have turned out disastrously and the resultant sense of responsibility or guilt was more than she could bear. Finally, some dependent parents may temporarily feel that they cannot cope with their child; rather than risk another mistake, they try to involve the teacher in future decisions. This type of dependency is rarely a persistent problem, because guilt, indecision, and feeling psychologically burdened are normal human emotions when they occur sporadically.

Excessively dependent parents are frightened. The teacher's task is not to heighten their anxiety by turning away from them but to gradually wean them away from their dependency. The parent's decisions and actions should be reinforced. When a parent asks for the teacher's opinion or when he is asked to help make a decision, statements such as the following might prove helpful:

> "I can appreciate that it's difficult to know what to do, but I don't think my opinion is any better than yours. What do you think should be done?"
> "That's a tough predicament. I'm not certain that I'd know what to do if I was faced with that situation. I'm wondering what your thoughts are?"

For the parent who insists that the teacher offer an opinion or make a decision:

> "It must feel like a difficult decision to make. I'd like to be of help as much as I can, but I really believe that people feel better about themselves when they make their own tough decisions, even if they don't always turn out right. I know I feel better when I do."

Teachers might be particularly susceptible to dependent parents. People in the helping professions thrive on the dependence or conferred authority others place on them; it allows them to do their job and meet their need to be helpful. Therefore, they can easily be seduced into a relationship with someone who has strong dependency needs.

OVERLY HELPFUL PARENTS

Helpful parents can be a real asset to the teacher, not only with their own children but also, on occasion, in the classroom. However, the *overly* helpful, energetic, and well-meaning parent, can become a challenge.

Excessively helpful parents are motivated by their need to be useful—a need that may not be satisfied in their other relationships. Overly helpful parents may have been praised in childhood when they contributed in some way to the family. Other such parents may have developed overfunctioning tendencies because of chronic illness in the family or an alcoholic parent who was needy and demanding. The major problem in the parent–teacher relationship is not so much the parent's desire to be helpful as it is the teacher's inability to communicate, in a sensitive way, that only a limited amount of assistance is needed. Parents generally understand clear, nonthreatening feedback from the teacher. Below are three ways a teacher may tell a parent that her assistance is appreciated yet more help than can be constructively used:

"Mrs. Greenwald, sometimes I don't know what I would do without you. You've been a tremendous help on numerous occasions. However, there are times when I feel things are very much in control, and there is little else to be done. I wonder if we can reduce the amount of time you spend with us and have you be 'on call' as the need arises. Does that seem like a workable solution to you?"

"I know you want to be helpful, and the kids really enjoy your involvement, but there are times when I feel that I don't need as much help as you are willing to offer. I very much appreciate your assistance, but a more reduced time schedule would work out better for me. How does that suit you?"

"I appreciate your comments about how I might work more effectively with Jason [the parent's son]. You have useful insights into teaching and classroom management. By your comments, however, I sometimes get the impression that you feel I should alter my way of doing things. Is my perception correct or am I off base?"

A comment such as the last one invites a dialogue between the two parties that often leads to some type of resolution.

OVERPROTECTIVE PARENTS

Overprotective parents are typically anxious about their child's welfare. They worry about his academic progress, yet their major concerns center around protection against physical or psychological harm. This behavior is often a reflection of being warned as children to be careful about accidents, disease, befriending certain peers, and the like, thus culminating in a fearful attitude about most things. Such parents are careful of what they eat and tend to be conservative in what they do. They worry and fret, and when something of concern to them occurs (which is just about everything), their anxiety increases and their fearfulness seems justified to them and is further reinforced.

Perhaps due to feelings of guilt, parents of children with disabilities may be particularly susceptible to overprotecting their children. Some may shield their child from tasks he is capable of performing successfully or from social interactions they consider harmful, such as situations in which he might be hurt physically.

The existentialists may have something to offer by way of explanation. They believe that the primary cause of man's anxiety is represented by the thin line between life and death (Yalom, 1980). Therefore, a type of low-key but pervasive anxiety about many situations is normal, and for most of us, anxiety is not relentless or unbearable. An existential psychologist might comment that overprotective parents have a heightened sense of their precarious existence and thus protect against tragedy by excessive care.

From another point of view, overprotection is seen as a compensatory behavior to make up for socially undesirable feelings, such as rejection; that is, overprotection is an exaggerated response to unacceptable negative feelings toward the child. Other parents feel that the existing disability must not be compounded by other difficulties. The child, they feel, is already significantly impaired, so that strenuous efforts must be exercised to minimize the possibility of other problems.

Often, overprotectiveness inhibits growth, as children are protected from a variety of situations which would otherwise expand their horizons and add to their knowledge and confidence. Overprotected children often develop fears not found among children who have been granted reasonable freedom within a loving family, thereby adding to and exacerbating the existing disability.

Overprotective parents are not likely to change their behavior easily, if at all. Nevertheless, the teacher owes it to the child and the family to suggest more realistic, growth-promoting practices. Whenever possible, independent actions initiated by the child should be reinforced so that he will continue the behavior. At conferences, the parents can be told of the child's gains, especially acquired skills or behaviors that facilitate independent thinking and living. The teacher might show her delight at these achievements and suggest activities that help develop the child's self-esteem and ability to cope. Some parents are so convinced that their child is impaired that they are pleasantly surprised to hear from the teacher or to see classroom achievements that they thought were impossible.

When parents seem unwilling to modify their overprotective behavior, which is clearly detrimental to the child, the teacher may wish to relate her observations in an unambiguous and firm fashion. For example:

"I think I understand your desire to help Lois and to protect her, but I wonder if it keeps her from certain growth-promoting experiences. Parents have a natural tendency to want to protect their children from harm, and it demonstrates their love and concern. This is good, but sometimes too much protection can keep a youngster from developing skills that she will need later in life and will help her to feel good about herself."

Overprotective parents who are particularly resistant to change are those whose needs are being met by such behavior. Unconsciously, the parents may wish to keep the child at an infantile level, enabling them to give and receive love and to feel useful. After all, an independent, virtually self-sufficient child is hardly gratifying to parents who require people to be dependent upon them. It is difficult for the teacher to exercise much leverage in this case. Also, as the parents' circumstances change, their sense of loneliness or lack of love from others may be gratified either in new, fulfilling relationships or in other ways.

NEGLECTFUL PARENTS

Nothing is more heartbreaking to a teacher than a child, clearly in need of love and proper care, who is barely attended to by his parents. They may be so preoccupied with other family members or problems that they cannot extend themselves further. They may reject the child because of his disability or because he was not wanted. (It is important to note that feelings of rejection can be expressed in at least two contradictory ways: overprotection due to intense guilt or outright neglect.)

In some instances, parents may equate neglect with independence, or neglect may be the consequence of their lifestyle, in which attending to their children is secondary to other pleasures or problems (e.g., alcoholism). In any event, child neglect is a serious problem of which the teacher must be aware. The circumstances surrounding neglect dictate the difficulties that might be expected. For example, the parent who mistakenly equates neglect with independence is quite different from the one who rejects the child or is preoccupied with major family problems that sometimes are exacerbated by poverty or illness.

In severe cases, it is advisable to inform the school social worker or other experienced authorities, who then attempt to work with the parents. In these instances, a referral to a children and youth service agency may be necessary. The social worker may ask the teacher about her observations of the child from time to time.

Other than informing the social worker and perhaps the principal, the teacher's recourse when she suspects that neglect is significant and long-standing is to help compensate to the extent possible for what the child is not receiving at home. The teacher can demonstrate concern for the neglected child both verbally and, on occasion, when appropriate, physically (a hug or pat on the back). The teacher can also set up situations in the classroom in which the child is included in group activities and occasionally assumes a position of leadership.

Neglectful parents resemble uncooperative parents except in one significant way: The latter generally provide the love, attention, and support the child needs at home. Neglectful parents, however, compound their lack of cooperation with school personnel by not providing the child with the essential emotional ingredients needed for healthy development.

Because parents who neglect their children are not motivated to cooperate with the teacher, access to these parents may be difficult. Sometimes the social worker can facilitate a parent–teacher meeting, but no matter how frustrating and unrewarding, the teacher should continue attempts to engage the parent. The possibility of a home visit should not be ruled out, if the parent appears willing.

Numerous efforts to involve the parents may eventually bear fruit. When this does occur, the teacher is confronted with the admittedly difficult task of what to say or do when the parent finally arrives at the conference. Incidentally, some neglectful parents routinely attend parent conferences, believing that in doing so, they have met their parental obligation.

In conferring with the parents, the teacher should avoid blaming them for the child's problems. Only when she believes the situation has grave consequences for the child, and the parents seem not to be aware of it or consciously continue to neglect the child, should she confront the issue in open, honest terms or report the neglect (or abuse) to the proper authorities. Before more drastic measures are taken, the teacher might point out to the parents the contrast in the child's response when he is attended to and when he is not. The child may thrive on positive attention of others and show discouragement and unruly behavior when he is ignored over sustained periods.

Incidents involving the withholding of food, adequate shelter, clothes, and love require a more direct approach. The teacher should make every attempt to make the parents cognizant of the impact neglect has on the child, even at the risk of offending them. However, I recommend that teachers confer with other school professionals before taking active measures. For some parents, a significant lack of parenting skills, combined with immaturity, can lead to problematic parent–child relationships. Because many parents could benefit from training and education in parenting skills, community agencies routinely offer parenting classes and workshops, often at little or no expense. A teacher may deal with damaging and intractable neglect by saying something like the following:

> "I realize that you face numerous problems at home, but Susie is just crying out for any signs of love she can get. Before the situation gets worse, to the point that your child needs more help than you and I can give her, I would urge you to try to let her know that you care."

> "I really feel uncomfortable commenting on Jerry's dress and behavior, but I believe that if I don't, no one will, and the situation will continue. I've been aware that Jerry comes to school disheveled most of the time. He doesn't seem to be getting enough to eat, and whenever another child has some candy, Jerry begs for some, or steals it. I've been wondering whether Jerry is ill or not getting enough food at home. He looks tired and frequently falls asleep in the classroom. Have you observed the same things, and if so, what do you think causes these things?"

Some of us have been witness to remarkably destructive relationships within families. Fortunately, child neglect, especially the neglect of children with disabilities, is not the norm, but it does exist. Nevertheless, as concerned outsiders, teachers must make every effort to be a positive influence in situations in which children are the victims of psychological or physical neglect or abuse. Sometimes other school personnel need to be involved; at other times, observations must be conveyed to parents in an open and direct way; in extreme cases, other agencies need to become involved.

PARENTS AS CLIENTS

Because of pressing personal problems, parents may seek the help of the teacher. Such problems may center around acute or chronic concerns related to the child with a disability, or they may range from transient feelings of frustration and anger over minor incidents to situations that severely threaten family integration (e.g., divorce).

Teachers, by engaging a colleague or friend to listen to a problem and, conversely, by offering help to a friend who needs a concerned ally, at different times have assumed the roles of both counselor and counselee. There is a great difference, however, between an empathic listener and a trained professional counselor or psychologist. This type of situation requires the teacher to make an important distinction about whether the parents need someone to empathize or be supportive, or someone who is trained to provide psychotherapy.

Temporary problems, which at the time appear to the parent to be significant but really constitute expected and easily resolved crises, can often be dealt with by the teacher. A parent's frustration over toilet training her child usually does not require psychological help. Often, concerns that appear bothersome but are temporary and not debilitating merely require the occasional presence of a concerned listener.

However, one needs to be cautious of situations in which parents, having significant problems, either overtly or covertly coax the teacher into the role of a professional counselor or psychotherapist. Teachers who are seen as warm and skilled interviewers, and who make themselves accessible to parents, are potentially attractive counselors. Having friends and parents come to a teacher for help because he is a good listener is an excellent endorsement for anyone in a people-oriented profession. However, teachers who are good listeners and convey a sense of caring must also be able to distinguish between major and minor problems that parents are experiencing. For the most part, a teacher's judgment improves with experience, but before discussing some cues to look for in significantly troubled parents, let us examine some of the reasons parents may look to teachers for counseling.

Some parents may seek help from their child's teacher because she is physically accessible. Others may not know where else to seek help. Parents may know of professional assistance but be confused by the array of titles (psychologist, psychiatrist, social worker, counselor) and wonder whether a certain type of professional may be more advantageous than another. In discussing different professional disciplines with parents, a teacher can provide a brief description of professionals' academic background and whatever other accurate information she happens to know about their professional training. Referrals should be based on the professional's reputation, including what is known about his ethical conduct, the personality "fit" with the parents, and the cost. Finally, parents may be reluctant to seek the help of a psychologist because of the stigma attached to doing so. Some people are greatly troubled by the implications of needing help for psychological problems, although, in some segments of society, having one's own therapist is a status symbol. If a referral is indicated and parents are open to it, professional societies (e.g., a state's Psychological Association) and medical schools are excellent sources of referral. Another good resource would be a professional recommended by a friend or colleague of the parents. It is generally wise for the teacher not to make a personal recommendation other than to an agency, hospital, or professional society.

Parents with the following complaints often require professional psychological assistance:

1. Deep and unrelenting depression and/or anxiety, which may be accompanied by insomnia, lack of concentration, or nightmares; suicidal thoughts might be expressed.
2. Strong feelings of rejection and accompanying guilt toward the child with a disability (a factor that may contribute to item 1).
3. Indications that family unity is being threatened (comments about significant and continuous arguments; discussion of impending separation and divorce or family violence, or substance abuse).
4. Comments about the considerable difficulty a nondisabled sibling has adjusting to the child with a disability.
5. Remarks suggesting severe neglect of the child or physical abuse.

6. Indications that the child with a disability is developing psychological problems, for example, depression, unexplained aggression.

Parents must be dissuaded from seeking a teacher's help in resolving any long-standing or significant problems. The teacher must communicate her concern over the parents' plight yet decline to assume a therapeutic role. She must make the parents aware that their problem(s) appear to need psychological attention and that she is not professionally prepared to be of assistance. If this fact is communicated sensitively and in a caring manner, parents may then be able to ask where professional help is available. (It is not uncommon for a recommendation to be acted upon months after a referral is suggested.)

The teacher should have at her disposal the names of community mental health agencies and professional organizations. (As noted earlier, private practice therapist referrals are best obtained through professional state societies.) Community clinics are generally less costly than engaging a private psychologist, but some people prefer a private practitioner. Professional counselors and psychotherapists with good reputations for dealing with families of children who have special needs are a particularly good resource to have available.

Parents who subtly imply or forcefully insist that the teacher provide the kind of help needed to resolve major problems might be informed that it would be improper for her to assume such a role:

"I get the feeling that you are asking me to help you with a problem for which I am not trained. I am really flattered that you trust me enough to confide in me, but because I can't really be of help to you, I'd like to suggest a few possibilities where you can get assistance from a trained professional. In any event, I'd like us to continue to schedule our parent conferences to discuss Joan's progress in school."

This comment communicates several important themes: The teacher is aware of the problem and the parents' desire to be helped by her; she knows her professional limitations but is concerned about the parents; she is willing to help the parents locate an appropriately trained professional; she wants to continue to meet with the parents, but she shifts the major focus of future meetings to the child.

FIGHTING PARENTS

As indicated, a number of authors have commented on the importance of having both parents at conferences, and this point cannot be over-emphasized. In this way, both parents and teacher are involved in planning for the child, and any differing perceptions or opinions are subject to examination during the meetings. In some situations, these conferences can challenge the interpersonal skills of the teacher more than any other meetings.

During conferences, the teacher should not look negatively upon parents who argue with each other. If nothing else, it allows the teacher to gain a fuller understanding of family dynamics, which may help to explain behavior not previously understood. Such parental interaction highlights conflicts that exist in the family and may be related to the psychological adjustment of both their child with a disability and nondisabled offspring.

Sometimes the teacher will find himself in the uncomfortable position of listening to a heated argument between parents and not knowing how or whether to intervene. Since this is an infrequent occurrence and is not the norm, discomfort with fighting parents is to be expected. There are, however, a few guidelines that the teacher might find helpful under these circumstances.

Teachers are not marriage counselors, and parents whose interactions suggest significant family problems should be referred to a qualified professional. The teacher should avoid involvement in heated arguments that symbolize deep-seated problems. Even highly qualified professionals find intervention during an animated exchange between family members a challenge. However, teachers may have individualized reactions to such conflict situations. Because of what teachers experienced as children with their families of origin, they will either have a high tolerance for conflict or very little. For example, some teachers have learned that arguments and conflict lead to bad outcomes; others have learned that conflict is a normal way of life and tends to strengthen, not weaken, relationships.

Some parental disagreements are mild and reflect an easily resolved difference of opinion. In some cases, the arguments may be the consequence of having partial information, or information that is perceived differently. Sometimes, the teacher can see that both parental perspectives are valid, and a sensitive comment can change a competitive situation to one of cooperation and understanding. For example, a teacher may respond as follows to a mother who feels that more emphasis should be placed on her child's appearance and social behavior and a father who values the importance of academic achievement:

> "In sitting here and listening to you, I can't help but agree with both of you. In looking to the future, Karen's behavior, appearance, and schoolwork will be important. I wonder if instead of concentrating on one or two of these concerns we can, without pushing Karen too much, work on all three. What would you think of a program that balances the three areas?"

When arguments are based on incomplete or inaccurate information, the teacher might comment:

> "I can understand that with the information you have been given, your confusion about whether Bobby will be able to go to college is growing. I'm not sure if this will help, but let's review and discuss the available information. According to his tested IQ score, Bobby should be able to compete successfully in college. What clouds the picture somewhat are the indications of specific learning disabilities that interfere with his learning now and, if not corrected, will interfere in college. Therefore, our efforts should be to correct, to the extent possible, the deficiencies we already know about, so that his learning will not be as frustrating for him in the future as it is now. If his motivation to go to college is high and we are able to decrease the impact of existing learning problems, Bobby should succeed in college. I don't know if this helps to make things clearer. Do you have any questions or thoughts?"

Whether parents are fighting over family concerns of some importance or arguing about an easily resolvable issue, the cardinal rule for the teacher is to avoid taking sides. If the teacher is to get involved at all, she should seek a compromise solution. She will have to contend with a most difficult problem if parents perceive that she favors one or the other of them. She needs to guard against the urge to intervene, especially when she privately does side with one of the parents.

Finally, teachers are sometimes shocked and frightened by parents who characteristically relate to each other in an animated fashion. What the teacher experiences during an emotional conference may run counter to her own experiences with her parents. Often, cultural factors play a role in how families interact. While families from some cultures communicate with considerable animation, others do so in more stoic, cerebral fashion. If parents interact in a manner contrary to the teacher's experience, it may cause some initial discomfort, but the discomfort should ease over time, especially when the teacher embraces the notion that a variety of family interactions are normal. During conferences, it is essential for the teacher to discriminate between the expression of major family problems, minor disagreements, and diverse styles of interpersonal interactions. Some family members deal with each other in a quiet, rational manner; others are more vocal and emotional. One style of interaction is not better or healthier than the other, just different.

INVOLVED–UNINVOLVED PARENTS

From time to time, teachers confront parents who say all the right things and convey a strong sense of cooperation during conferences yet fail to carry out agreed-upon courses of action. Such behavior can be confusing and frustrating for the teacher, but an examination of the possible motives behind it should prove helpful.

As with the other challenging parents, the reasons for observable behavior differ from parent to parent. For example, two parents may differ in how they discipline their children. One might be motivated to be strict because that was how he was raised. The other parent may have been basically raised in the same way but feels that overly strict parent tends to reinforce anxiety in children. Some behaviors are multidetermined; that is, more than one causal factor contributes to a specific behavior.

A parent's wish to please the teacher or other school personnel with her positive intentions and general willingness to be cooperative may account for her behavior. She may feel that she has to convey interest so that her child will continue to be accepted in the program or school, or so that the teacher will view both the parents and the child in a positive way. Some parents genuinely want to be helpful and cooperative, and have every intention of pursuing activities decided upon in collaboration with the teacher, but somehow they find these actions impossible to initiate. For some parents, the demands of other members of the family and work may be so great that good intentions are difficult to implement. For others, engaging in mutually agreed-upon activities with their child serves to highlight their child's deficiencies, thereby increasing their anxiety and subsequent withdrawal.

Although they may agree with the teacher that certain activities should be undertaken at home, some parents may actually feel that these home activities fall within the scope of the classroom. Such parents resent engaging in activities they feel the teacher is trained to conduct and should carry out in school. Other parents think they cannot adequately perform the tasks agreed upon and, therefore, will not risk failure or harm to the child; some parents characteristically agree to complete a task, then fail to do so. Still others are chronic procrastinators and never catch up.

Discovering what lies behind parents' failure requires sensitivity and tact. The teacher must be sure that his own frustration and anger do not become an impediment to effective communication. He must not blame the parents for the child's slow progress or imply that they are liars, lack responsibility, or are untrustworthy. It does little good to point out the discrepancy between what the parents said they would do and what they actually do. However, in some situations the teacher must find some way of communicating his concern to the parent.

> "I know it must be difficult at times with the other responsibilities you have, but if one of you could spend about one-half hour, three times a week with Joan in a reading activity, I believe it would help her retain whatever gains she has made in school."

> "I'm sure it must be hard to be reminded constantly of the things Jimmy does not do well, and it must be frustrating to have him do things over and over again, with little to show for it, but I believe that if we work together and are consistent with him at home and at school, he will begin to make small gains. It's discouraging not to see more progress, yet I feel that some progress has been made and that more is possible, but I very much need your help. What do you think—can we work together on this?"

In both responses, the teacher recognizes the parents' underlying feelings (of frustration and discouragement), which tells them that he is trying to understand their problems. In the first response, the teacher describes the advantages of having academic activities reinforced at home. Also, he depicts the demands on the parents' time as modest and shared, so that working with the child is not seen as overwhelming. In the second response, parental feelings are again recognized and communicated. Also, the parents are asked to become allies with the teacher in the interest of their child. The teacher takes an optimistic view of past gains and future achievements, without promising significant and unrealistic progress. Finally, the parents are asked how they feel about the teacher's comments.

In contrast, responses that would probably result in increased resistance may resemble the following:

Teacher 1: "Mrs. Allen, I don't know how many times I've asked you to positively reinforce John whenever he goes to the bathroom. Unless you do what I keep telling you to do, John may never be toilet trained. What's the matter, don't you care enough about your son to do this little thing that I ask?"

Teacher 2: "I don't know what's going on at home, but I just don't understand what is keeping you from being more consistent with Leslie. It's really a very simple thing that I'm asking you to do. The next time we meet, I hope to hear that you are working consistently with Leslie."

Teacher 3: "I'm getting tired of hearing about all the great activities you promise to do with Scott but never carry out. It's time now to take some action on what you say you are going to do."

These responses—examples of cajoling, rudeness, and threats—can easily lead to guilt, defensiveness, and hostility, which, unfortunately, will take their toll on the parent–teacher relationship and the child. The teacher appears uninterested in the reasons for the parents' behavior or their emotions, and he converts his own impotent and angry feelings into a scolding.

Parents who believe that learning activities should take place only in a classroom may change their minds if a teacher takes the time to explain how gains made at school can be reinforced at home to benefit their child. These parents may need to know that additional help at home is particularly important for children with disabilities and that many parents now work with their children in collaboration with the teacher. This last point can be construed as an attempt to apply pressure on parents, but it gives them a perspective on contemporary home–school relationships.

Parents who feel they cannot successfully work with their children might be willing to try if the demands are not too great and if they have success, thereby increasing their self-confidence. It may be helpful for the parents to understand that they cannot harm the child through home activities. However, parents who are too anxious to work with their child at home or are currently too burdened to effectively help should never be pressured to do so.

ETHICAL CONCERNS

Contrary to what some people believe, ethics refer more to issues of professional judgment than to legalistic implications, although a breach of ethics can lead to legal problems. Personal judgment (good sense) and judgment based on ethical codes of conduct developed by professional societies (e.g., the National Education Association) should guide teachers' behavior.

The ethical issue of confidentiality is important to professionals regardless of their professional affiliation. In this regard, teachers must be careful about who is privy to confidential information and who is not. Breaches of confidentiality can be detrimental to both children and parents, as well as to the teacher, and certainly to the parent–teacher relationship. Confidential breaches tend to occur most often under two circumstances: (1) when the teacher is angry at a child or parent and seeks revenge, or (2) when the teacher is unaware of the circumstances under which confidential information should not be shared.

All professionals encounter parents or clients who provide significant challenges. Some parents take up inordinate amounts of time and energy or are constantly complaining about some facet of their child's education. As a consequence, they generate feelings of frustration, anger, or anxiety in the teacher. For the teacher, a natural and often a helpful tendency under such conditions is to vent her feelings to a member of her own family, a friend, or a colleague. Little harm is done in discussing, *in a general way,* a frustrating situation, but the discussion must avoid content that would in any way identify the parent. Such discussions are safer with a professional colleague or supervisor, where confidentiality is less of an issue and the teacher can openly express her feelings and also be in a position to receive helpful feedback. Breaches of confidential information to friends and acquaintances are a serious matter that raise questions of appropriate professional conduct.

Information shared between parent and teacher must remain private unless other involved professionals in the school (e.g., school social worker) are consulted. Test and/or anecdotal information retained in files is likewise considered confidential to uninvolved professionals, as well as to people outside of the school. Consultants and other professionals may have access to confidential information only if the parent signs a release-of-information form. In such instances, parents should be fully informed as to who will have access to the information and for what purposes.

Legislation makes it mandatory that parents have available to them information about their child. This enables parents to examine information that was not previously available to them and to respond to any inaccuracies found in the files. It also is incumbent upon those making file entries to consider carefully and accurately report any information about the child and parent.

As mentioned earlier, the use of recording devices for supervision purposes should only be used when the parent has been informed of the recording, the reason for it, who will be listening to it, and how it will be used. The only legitimate reason for recording parent–teacher conferences is for learning purposes, and not under any circumstances for the collection of "evidence."

Performing activities in a professional manner generally ascribed to one's role is an ethical matter. Subsumed in this category is a commitment to work as effectively as possible with children and parents. Using principles of good interpersonal relationships is important, as is making oneself accessible to parents. In general, the teacher owes it to himself and the children and parents he serves to take his job seriously, with dedication and enthusiasm, even though at times his level of motivation may be low. It is a serious concern if a teacher's interest and motivation wane significantly, since the teaching profession, with its challenges, requires the services of people with high principles, motivation, interest, and knowledge.

When teachers are not sure of the propriety of their actions, they often find it helpful to consult the code of ethical standards developed by the professional organization to which they belong. Such codes have been prepared for the specific purpose of providing guidance to the professional.

TEACHER BURNOUT

The diverse and sometimes contradictory demands placed upon teachers can, over extended periods of time, lead to what has in other professions become a recognized phenomenon: professional burnout. Burnout has become a particularly critical issue not only in the mental health profession but also in medicine and other professions where high levels of sustained stress can result in anger, frustration, discouragement, loss of control, loss of confidence, and so forth.

The seeds of disillusionment are sown during the teacher's experiences in college. Students are taught the high ideals they should bring to their chosen profession—ideals that tend to become tarnished in the day-to-day encounters with students, supervisors, and parents. Educators of teachers must be more aware of the significant gap between these ideals and reality, a major source of disappointment to novice teachers. Also, some professors who talk about the importance of productive interpersonal relationships are themselves distant, closed, and manipulative in their contacts with their students—hardly a proper social model for students who look to their professors for guidance that is often accomplished through emulation.

Disillusionment grows in the realities of the job. Teachers are often confronted with high demands and low rewards. Each day brings its quota of problems, from students who lack the motivation for learning to parents who are critical. In many classrooms, high student–teacher ratios and discipline problems allow little opportunity for more personal relationships between student and teacher. It is of some consequence to note that the selection of a people-oriented profession is motivated by a need for close interpersonal relationships that can be frustrated in certain school environments.

Positive feedback from students and parents, a major source of fulfillment, is intermittent and, therefore, not particularly reinforcing. This situation, coupled with the lack of reinforcement from supervisors and administrators, can be discouraging. Teachers' professional esteem may further erode as they are asked to assume new roles and implement new school policies and mandated laws.

Sooner or later, teachers may become exhausted to the point that they no longer look forward with anticipation and excitement to their work. The following recommendations are offered to help prevent burnout:

1. School administrators should have opportunities to teach, so that they are in a better position to empathize with the teacher.
2. Teachers should be given greater voice in the formulation of policy. At minimum, they should be given opportunities (e.g., in faculty meetings) to voice their opinions, no matter how unpopular, and be guaranteed that their comments will not be held against them. Having a voice in one's destiny is an important builder of morale.
3. Schools should make provisions for teachers to spend time away from the classroom during the school year. For example, teachers should be relieved periodically for a period of time to

pursue other activities or hobbies. These minisabbaticals often provide an opportunity for renewal. At the very least, they give teachers the impression that the system, which is often viewed as an adversary, is concerned about their welfare.

4. Teachers should have opportunities to suggest areas in which they feel deficient, so that in-service training programs can be built around their perceived needs. This input should greatly increase teachers' interest and motivation to attend such programs.

5. It is perhaps a radical idea, but schools should make available for teachers support groups where concerns, gripes, and professionally related problems can be aired. Such meetings can relieve some of the tension that may exist in the school.

Resources to Help Teachers Help Parents

Compiled by Karen Seligman, MEd

Parents of children with disabilities sometimes need help to resolve acute personal crises as well as long-term problems. At other times, parents may need concrete information, inspiration, support, and insight. The following resources have been developed so that teachers may have available to them referral sources and reading materials to serve better the parents with whom they work.

It should be noted that the lists of agencies and references in this appendix are far from complete. The reader should supplement these lists with other useful references and resources that exist in the teacher's community. All reading material recommended to parents, whether referred to in this Appendix or not, ought to be reviewed by the teacher. Also, before recommending readings and making referrals to agencies, teachers should be knowledgeable about the parents, so that their recommendations are appropriate.

SOCIAL SERVICE AGENCIES

Arthritis

Arthritis Foundation
1330 West Peachtree Street
Atlanta, GA 30309
800-283-7800 or 404-872-7100
FAX: 404-872-0457

Seeks to discover the cause and improve the methods of treatment and prevention of arthritis and other rheumatic diseases.

Autism

Autism Society of America
7910 Woodmont Avenue, Suite 650
Bethesda, MD 20814
301-657-0881 or 800-3-AUTISM
FAX: 301-657-0869

Informs the public of the symptoms and problems of children and adults with autism.

Autism Network International
PO Box 448
Syracuse, NY 13210-0448
e-mail: jisincla@mailbox.syr.edu

Self-help and advocacy organization for autistic individuals.

Blindness

American Foundation for the Blind
11 Penn Plaza, Suite 300
New York, NY 10001
212-502-7600 or 800-232-5463
FAX: 212-502-7777
TDD: 212-502-7662
e-mail: afbinfo@afb.org

Provides information and referral service.

American Printing House for the Blind
1839 Frankfort Avenue
PO Box 6085
Louisville, KY 40206-0085
502-895-2405 or 800-223-1839
FAX: 502-899-2274
e-mail: info@aph.org

Produces literature in all media for the blind. Manufactures educational aids for use by visually impaired persons.

American Council of the Blind
1155 15th Street, NW, Suite 720
Washington, DC 20005
202-467-5081 or 800-424-8666
FAX: 202-467-5085

Serves as a national clearinghouse on blindness for individuals, organizations, and institutions.

National Association for Visually Handicapped
22 West 21st Street
New York, NY 10010
212-889-3141
FAX: 212-727-2931
e-mail: staff@navh.org

Acts as information clearinghouse for public and private services available to the partially seeing. Offers guidance and counseling to adults and parents of partially seeing children.

Cancer

American Cancer Society
1599 Clifton Road, NE
Atlanta, GA 30329
404-320-3333 or 800-ACS-2345
FAX: 404-329-7530

A volunteer organization supporting education and research in cancer prevention, diagnosis, detection, and treatment.

Cancer Care
1180 Avenue of the Americas
New York, NY 10036
212-221-3300 or 212-719-0263

Promotes and aids the development of social services to patients and families stricken by cancer throughout the United States and worldwide.

Candlelighters Childhood Cancer Foundation
7910 Woodmont Avenue, Suite 460
Bethesda, MD 20614-3015
301-657-8401 or 800-366-2224
FAX: 301-718-2686
Website: http://www.candlelighters.org
e-mail: Info@candlelighters.org

Educates, supports, serves, and advocates for families and individuals touched
by childhood cancer.

Cerebral Palsy

United Cerebral Palsy Association
1660 L Street, NW, Suite 700
Washington, DC 20036-5602
800-872-5827 or 800-USA-5UCP or 202-776-0406
FAX: 202-776-0414

Provides advocacy and information, and promotes medical research.

Communication Disorders

National Association for Hearing and Speech Action
10801 Rockville Pike
Rockville, MD 20852
301-897-8682 or 800-638-8255
FAX: 301-571-0457
e-mail: irc@asha.org

Provides educational and referral information on speech, language, and hearing disabilities.

Cystic Fibrosis (*See also* Respiratory Disorders)

Cystic Fibrosis
6931 Arlington Road, Suite 200
Bethesda, MD 20814
301-951-4422 or 800-344-4823
FAX: 301-951-6378

Supports medical research, professional education, and care centers to benefit
patients with cystic fibrosis.

Deafness

National Institute on Deafness and Other Communication Disorders
One Communications Avenue
Bethesda, MD 20892-3456
800-241-1044
FAX: 301-907-8830
TDD: 800-241-1055

Disseminates information on normal and disordered processes relating to hearing, balance, smell, taste, voice, speech, and language.

National Information Center on Deafness (NICD)
800 Florida Avenue, NE
Washington, DC 20002
202-651-5051 or 202-651-5052
FAX: 202-651-5054
TDD: 202-651-5052
e-mail: nicd@gallux.gallaudet.edu

Provides information on deafness for professionals and the public.

National Association of the Deaf
814 Thayer Avenue, Suite 250
Silver Springs, MD 20910-4500
301-587-1788 (voice) or 301-587-1789
FAX: 301-587-1791
Website: www.nad.org
e-mail: nadhq@juno.com

An association for adult deaf persons, parents of deaf children, professionals, students in the field of deafness, and other interested individuals.

Diabetes

National Diabetes Information Clearinghouse
One Information Way
Bethesda, MD 20892-3560
301-654-3327
FAX: 301-907-8906

Information and referral service of the National Institute of Diabetes and Digestive and Kidney Diseases. Provides referrals, publications, support groups, and educational materials.

Juvenile Diabetes Foundation International
120 Wall Street
New York, NY 10005-3904
212-785-9500 or 800-JDF-CURE
FAX: 212-725-9595
e-mail: jbroch@jdf.usa.com

Supports juvenile diabetics and their families.

Epilepsy

Epilepsy Foundation of America
4351 Garden City Drive
Landover, MD 20785
301-459-3700 or 800-EFA-1000
FAX: 301-577-2684
e-mail: postmaster@eaf.org

Supports medical, social, rehabilitation, legal, employment, information, education, and advocacy programs.

Heart Disease

American Heart Association
7272 Greenville Avenue
Dallas, TX 75231-4596
214-373-6300 or 800-242-1793
FAX: 214-987-4334

Supports research, education, and community service programs.

Hemophilia

National Hemophilia Foundation
116 West 32nd Street, 11th Floor
New York, NY 10001
212-328-3700
FAX: 212-328-7777

Supports research, disseminates literature, conducts educational programs, and provides referrals.

Learning Disabilities

Learning Disabilities Association of America
4156 Library Road
Pittsburgh, PA 15234
412-341-1515 or 412-341-8077
TTY: 412-341-8077
FAX: 412-344-0224
e-mail: Idanatl@usaor.net

An alliance of professionals and parents of children with learning disabilities. Offers free information packet, counseling, education, and referral.

International Dyslexia Association
Chester Building, Suite 382
8600 La Salle Road
Baltimore, MD 21286-2044
410-296-0232 or 800-ABCD-123
FAX: 410-321-5069

Offers free information to the public and provides referrals for diagnosis and treatment.

Leukemia

Children's Leukemia Research Association
585 Stewart Avenue, Suite 536
Garden City, NY 11530
516-222-1944
FAX: 516-222-0457

Promotes research and public awareness. Provides referrals and financial aid to leukemia patients and their families.

Leukemia Society of America
600 Third Avenue
New York, NY 10016
212-573-8484 or 800-955-4LSA
FAX: 212-856-9686

Raises funds and conducts research, sponsors medical symposia, and provides financial aid and free information.

Mental Illness

National Alliance for the Mentally Ill
200 North Glebe Road, Suite 1015
Arlington, VA 22203-3754
703-524-7600 or 800-950-NAMI
FAX: 703-524-9094
e-mail: vanessa@nami.org

A self-help organization supporting advocacy, legislation, and family support groups. Provides information and referral services.

Mental Retardation

American Association on Mental Retardation
444 North Capitol Street, NW, Suite 846
Washington, DC 20001-1512
202-387-1968 or 800-424-3688
FAX: 202-387-2193

Interdisciplinary association of professionals and concerned individuals in the field. Works to promote the well-being of those with mental retardation. Publications, newsletters, and journals are available.

Association for Retarded Citizens
500 East Border Street, Suite 300
Arlington, TX 76010
817-261-6003
FAX: 817-277-3491
e-mail: thearc@metvonet.com

Parents, professional workers, and others interested in individuals with mental retardation. States have local associations of ARC that provide information and services.

Miscellaneous

Association for Persons with Severe Handicaps (TASH)
29 West Susquehanna Avenue, Suite 210
Baltimore, MD 21204-5201
410-828-8274
FAX: 410-828-6706
TDD: 410-828-1306

A group of professionals and family members that advocate on behalf of all persons with disabilities.

National Center for Youth with Disabilities
University of Minnesota, Box 21
420 Delaware Street, Southeast
Minneapolis, MN 55455
612-626-2825
FAX: 612-626-2134
e-mail: ncyd.@gold.tc.umn.edu

Information and resource center focusing on adolescents with chronic illnesses
and disabilities and their transition to adult life. NCYD also maintains the National Resource Library and a database of information. Publications are available.

National Lekotek Center
2100 Ridge Avenue
Evanston, IL 60201-2796
708-328-0001 or 800-366-7529
FAX: 708-328-5514

Fosters the inclusion of children with disabilities into family and community
activities through play-based programs.

Parents Helping Parents
3041 Olcott Street
Santa Clara, CA 95054-3222
408-727-5775
FAX: 408-727-0182

Resource center assists children with special needs. Offers training to parents
and professionals.

National Easter Seal Society
230 West Monroe Street, Suite 1800
Chicago, IL 60606-4802
312-726-6200 or 800-221-6827
TDD: 312-726-4258
FAX: 312-726-1494
e-mail: NESSinfo@seals.com

National charitable agency devoted to helping families and service providers.
Chapters exist in all states.

Family Service America, Inc.
11700 West Lake Park Drive
Milwaukee, WI 53224
414-359-1040 or 800-221-2681
FAX: 414-359-1074

Network of community-based, family counseling, and support services in
North America. Publishes a Directory of Member Organizations.

National Directory of Children, Youth, and Family Services
PO Box 1837
Longmont, CO 80502-1837
303-776-7539 or 800-343-6681
FAX: 303-776-5831

A guide to human social service agencies, health services, juvenile justice
agencies, and related service organizations, both local and nationwide.

National Information Center for Children and Youth with Disabilities
PO Box 1492
Washington, DC 20013
202-884-8200 or 800-695-0285
FAX: 202-884-8441

A national agency for families and professionals looking for information and
referrals for children and youth with disabilities.

American Association for Marriage and Family Therapy
1133 15th Street, NW, Suite 300
Washington, DC 20005-2710
202-452-0109 or 800-374-AMFT
FAX: 202-223-2329
e-mail: webmgr@aamft.org

Professional society of marriage and family therapists.

Association of Jewish Family and Children's Agencies
3086 Highway 27, Suite 11
PO Box 248
Kendall Park, NJ 08824-0248
908-821-0909 or 800-634-7346
FAX: 908-821-0493
e-mail: ajfca@aol.com

Provides services to families and children in the United States and Canada.
Publishes annual directory.

Multiple Sclerosis

National Multiple Sclerosis Society
733 Third Avenue
New York, NY 10017
212-986-3240 or 800-FIGHT-MS
FAX: 212-986-7981

Supports research and provides services for persons with multiple sclerosis.

Muscular Dystrophy

Muscular Dystrophy Association
3300 East Sunrise Drive
Tucson, AZ 85718
520-529-2000
FAX: 520-529-5300

Fosters research into the cause and cure of neuromuscular diseases.

Myasthenia Gravis

Myasthenia Gravis Foundation
1820 South 75th Street, Suite 120
West Allis, WI 53214
312-258-0522 or 800-541-5454 or 414-938-9800
FAX: 312-258-0461

Raises funds for research and for professional and public education programs.

Neurofibromatosis

National Neurofibromatosis Foundation
95 Pine Street
New York, NY 10005
212-344-6633 or 800-323-7938
FAX: 212-529-6094
Website: http://www.nf.org
e-mail: nnf@aol.com

Sponsors and conducts research, promotes clinical activities for patients, provides support services to patients and their families, and educates the public.

Osteogenesis Imperfecta

Osteogenesis Imperfecta Foundation
804 West Diamond Avenue, Suite 210
Gaithersburg, MD 20878
301-947-0083 or 800-981-2663
Website: http://www.oif.org
e-mail: bonelink@aol.com

Supports and encourages medical research, educates the public, and disseminates information to patients, their families, and medical professions.

Paraplegia

National Spinal Cord Injury Association
545 Concord Avenue, Suite 29
Cambridge, MA 02138-1122
800-962-9629
FAX: 617-441-3449
e-mail: nscia@aol.com

Seeks to inform and educate families and medical and allied professions about
persons with spinal cord injury and disease.

Spinal Cord Society
Wendell Road
Fergus Falls, MN 56537
218-739-5252
FAX: 218-739-5262

Promotes research and increases public awareness of issues pertaining to spinal cord injuries.

Prader–Willi Syndrome

Prader–Willi Syndrome Association U.S.A.
5700 Midnight Pass Road, Suite 6
Sarasota, FL 34242
941-312-0400 or 926-4797
FAX: 941-312-0142
Website: http://www.pwsausa.org
e-mail: pwsausa@aol.com

Works to provide a forum for communication about the syndrome, particularly the means to cope with it. Promotes research and the establishment of treatment facilities.

Respiratory Disorders

American Lung Association
1740 Broadway
New York, NY 10019-4374
212-315-8700
FAX: 212-265-5642
e-mail: info@lungusa.org

Works with other organizations in planning and conducting programs in community services, education, and research.

Spina Bifida

Spina Bifida Association of America
4590 MacArthur Boulevard, NW, Suite 250
Washington, DC 20007-4226
202-944-3285 or 800-621-3141
FAX: 202-944-3295

Provides information and promotes public awareness, conducts research, monitors the development of legislation, provides referral services, and seeks to improve vocational training of individuals with spina bifida.

Tay–Sachs Disease

National Tay–Sachs and Allied Diseases Association
2001 Beacon Street
Brookline, MA 02146
617-277-4463 or 800-906-8723
FAX: 617-277-0134
Website: http://mcrcr.med.nyu.edu/~murphp01/taysachs.htm
e-mail: NTSAD-Boston@worldnet.att.net

Supports education, prevention, and research. Provides literature, referrals, and offers support groups and services.

Tourette Syndrome

Tourette Syndrome Association
42-40 Bell Boulevard
Bayside, NY 11361
718-224-2999 or 800-237-0717
FAX: 718-279-9596
Website: http://TSA.mgh.harvard.edu
e-mail: tourette@ix.netcom.com

Develops and disseminates educational materials; stimulates support for research; apprises members of rights, services, and benefits provided by government and other organizations. Provides lists of experienced doctors; operates support groups and other services.

BOOKS FOR PARENTS

Raising a Child Who Has a Physical Disability
Donna G. Albrecht
John Wiley & Sons, Inc. (1995)

Topics include building a medical team, day-to-day coping, hospitalizations, clothing, and long-range planning.

Brothers and Sisters—A Special Part of Exceptional Families
Thomas H. Powell and Peggy Ahrenhold Gallagher
Paul H. Brookes Publishing Co. (1993)

A book for professionals and parents that includes information about sibling relationships, especially when one of the siblings has a disability. This book comprehensively covers the many areas of sibling life.

Deaf Like Me
Thomas S. Spradley and James P. Spradley
Gallaudet University Press (1987)

A father's story of one family's journey toward understanding deafness and embracing signing as a means of communication for their 5-year-old daughter.

Life As We Know It
Michael Bérubé
Vintage Books (1996)

A father describes the first 4 years of life with his son who has Down syndrome.

Babies with Down Syndrome
Karen Stray-Gundersen
Woodbine House (1995)

Details baby care, developmental issues, educational issues, and legal rights.

A Slant of Sun: One Child's Courage
Beth Kephart
W. W. Norton & Co. (1998)

The author describes her son's gradual emergence from a world of obsessive play rituals to enjoying others and building relationships.

Children with Cerebral Palsy: A Parent's Guide
Elaine Geralis
Woodbine House (1998)

This book provides information concerning medical issues, therapy, development, family life, schooling, goal setting, and advocacy.

Siblings of Children with Autism: A Guide for Families
Sandra L. Harris
Woodbine House (1994)

Chapters describe sibling relationships, how to explain autism to children, how to help children play, and family dynamics.

Friendships in the Dark
Phyllis Campbell
St. Martin's Paperbooks (1996)

A blind woman's story of the people and pets who light up her world.

Another Season
Gene Stallings and Sally Cook
Broadway Books (1997)

A football coach's story of raising an exceptional son.

Planet of the Blind: A Memoir
Stephen Kuusisto
Dial Press (1998)

The autobiography of a man who was born blind.

Why Johnny Can't Concentrate
Robert A. Moss, with Helen Huff Dunlap
Bantam Books (1990)

Coping with attention deficit disorder.

The Silent Garden: Raising Your Deaf Child
Paul W. Ogden
Gallaudet University Press (1996)

Provides parents of deaf children with information on the possibilities offered to deaf children today.

Portraying Persons with Disabilities: An Annotated Bibliography
    of Nonfiction for Children and Teenagers.
Joan Brest Friedberg, June B. Mullins, and Adelaide Weir Sukiennik
R. R. Bowker (1992)

Brief descriptions and evaluations of nonfiction books for children and adolescents.

A Guide to Understanding and Living with Epilepsy
Orrin Devinsky
F. A. Davis Co. (1994)

Topics include explaining epilepsy, drug and other therapies, how to obtain good medical care, and information about the American's with Disabilities Act.

Differences in Common: Straight Talk on Mental Retardation, Down Syndrome,
    and Life
Marilyn Trainer
Woodbine House (1991)

The challenges, joys, setbacks, and triumphs of coping with a child with Down syndrome.

*Special Children, Challenged Parents: The Struggles and Rewards of Raising
   a Child with a Disability*
Robert A. Naseef
Birch Lane Press (1997)

A moving account of the dynamics, challenges, and triumphs of families coping with childhood disability. Written from a father's perspective.

Uncommon Fathers: Reflections on Raising a Child with a Disability
Donald J. Meyer
Woodbine House (1995)

Essays written by fathers from all walks of life about their experiences with
their children who have disabilities.

A Difference in the Family
Helen Featherstone
Basic Books (1980)

A classic. Featherstone writes about the effects of childhood disability on the
family from the perspective of a mother and educator. Brilliantly written.

Epilepsy and the Family
Richard Lechtenberg
Harvard University Press (1984)

Covers adults and children with epilepsy, marital problems, sexual activity,
sibling issues, treatment issues, and the like.

Your Child Has a Disability: A Complete Sourcebook of Daily and Medical Care
Mark Batshaw
Paul H. Brookes Publishing Co. (1998)

Chock-full of medical, practical, and psychosocial information about most
childhood disabilities.

Cognitive Coping, Families, and Disability
Ann P. Turnbull, Joan M. Patterson, Shirley K. Behr, Douglas L. Murphy,
   Janet G. Marquis, and Martha J. Blue-Banning (Eds.)
Paul H. Brookes Publishing Co. (1993)

Positive approaches to help families cope and adjust to childhood disability.

Imagining Robert: My Brother, Madness, and Survival: A Memoir
Jay Neugeboren
William Morrow & Co., Inc. (1997)

Memoir of an established writer's relationship with a brother who has suffered the ravages of mental illness.

My Sister's Keeper: Learning to Cope with a Sibling's Mental Health
Margaret Moorman
Penguin Books (1993)

A poignant memoir of Moorman's struggle to come to grips with her sister's schizophrenia.

BOOKS FOR KIDS

Mom's Best Friend
Sally Hobart Alexander
Macmillan Publishing Co. (1992)

Describes, from a child's perspective, and with plenty of pictures, the adventures of a mother who is obtaining her next seeing-eye dog. Hobart Alexander is a blind author.

Taking Diabetes to School
Kim Gosselin
Joy Jo Books, LLC (1998)

A young boy describes how he lives with diabetes.

Kids Explore the Gifts of Children with Special Needs
Westridge Young Writers Workshop
John Muir Publications (1994)

Written by kids, in grades three through six, about students with disabilities.

Braille for the Sighted
Designed and illustrated by Jane Schneider and Kathy Kifer
Garlic Press (1998)

A book for seeing children interested in learning how to sight-read braille.

I Have a Sister: My Sister Is Deaf
Jeanne Whitehouse Peterson
HarperCollins (1977)

A book for young readers that describes a child's view of her deaf sister.

Andy and His Yellow Frisbee
Mary Thompson
Woodbine House (1996)

This book introduces young readers to autism.

Living with a Brother or Sister with Special Needs: A Book for Sibs
Donald J. Meyer, Patricia F. Vadasy, and Rebecca R. Fewell
University of Washington Press (1985)

A sensitive and down-to-earth book that addresses the many questions siblings have about their brother or sister with a disability.

Views from Our Shoes
Donald J. Meyer
Woodbine House (1997)

Forty-five siblings share their experiences of being a brother or sister of a child with a disability. These are short essays from siblings whose ages range from 4 to 18.

Listen for the Bus: David's Story
Patricia McMahon and John Godt
Boyds Mills (1995)

Readers are alerted to the many things David can do, while they are sensitized to his inability to see and his difficulty in hearing.

Someone Special, Just Like You
Tricia Brown and Fran Ortiz
Henry Holt & Co., Inc. (1995)

Portrays preschool disabled children actively playing and learning.

Seeing Things My Way
Carol S. Carter, Alden R. Carter, Alden S. Carter, and Abby Levine
Albert Whitman & Co. (1998)

With the help of special equipment and teachers, Amanda, who cannot see well, has fun and learns with her classmates.

Portraying Persons with Disabilities: An Annotated Bibliography of Nonfiction
   for Children and Teenagers
Joan Brest Friedberg, June B. Mullins, and Adelaide Weir Sukiennik
R. R. Bowker (1992)

This sourcebook provides information and a critical analysis of books written about persons with disabilities. The book selections were guided by eight criteria, including the selection of works that foster acceptance and understanding. Grade levels are given to help the reader make appropriate judgments regarding suitability. The compilers do state that the assignment of reading levels is subjective and should be flexibly applied given the reading acumen and maturity of the child reader. Nonetheless, the reading levels are a helpful guide for teachers, parents, and children.

The following is a sample of books reviewed by Friedberg, Mullins, and Sukiennik:

They Never Want to Tell You: Children Talk about Cancer
David J. Bearison
Harvard University Press (1991)

For grades 7–12. Eight children, ages 3–19, tell what it is like to have cancer. Introduction instructs adults in how to discuss cancer with children. The author is a professor in developmental psychology.

I Want to Grow Hair, I Want to Grow Up, I Want to Go to Boise:
   Children Surviving Cancer
Erma Bombeck
Harper & Row (1989)

For grades 9–12. Nationally known author and humorist, Erma Bombeck, has written a book about how children cope with cancer. In the book, she uses quotes, narrative, and pictures from children as they describe the realities of living with cancer.

Carnal Acts
Nancy Mairs
HarperCollins (1990)

For grades 10–12. Well-known author writes about the effect multiple sclerosis has had on her career, her thinking, her family, and her relationships. She writes compellingly of her disease and how she copes with it.

My Sister's Special
Jo Prall
Children's Press (1985)

For grades 1–3. A young boy writes about family life with his sister who has cerebral palsy and is mentally retarded. His positive outlook of his sister is reflected in both words and photographs.

Hellen Keller
Nigel Hunter
Bookwright (1986)

For grades 2–6. Although both deaf and blind, the author presents Keller as a courageous and happy person who went on to great achievements in her life.

Hellen Keller: A Light for the Blind
Kathleen V. Kudlinsky
Viking Press (1989)

For grades 4–6. Another book about this remarkable person by Kathleen Kudlinsky, who covers Keller's entire life, from her illness to her death at 87.

Finding a Common Language: Children Living with Deafness
Thomas Bergman
Gareth Stevens (1989)

For grades K–4. A story about a 6-year-old Swedish girl who has been deaf since birth. This illustrated book emphasizes the similarities of the deaf child and hearing children.

Beethoven
Alan Blackwood
Bookwright (1987)

For grades 4–6. Simple, well-written account of Beethoven's life and his ability to compose renowned music even after he became deaf.

A Child Called Noah
Josh Greenfield
Henry Holt & Co., Inc. (1986)

For grades 10–12. Hollywood writer, Josh Greenfield, chronicles his life with his son, Noah, and his family. Noah suffers from mental illness, which contributes to significant challenges for the family.

My Sister Is Special
Larry Jansen
Standard (1984)

For grades PS–1. The author has written this book in the voice of his son describing life with his younger sister who has Down syndrome. The book illustrates how a child can see his sister's special qualities along with characteristics that all humans exhibit.

Women Who Made a Difference
Malcolm Forbes and Jeff Block
Simon & Schuster, Inc. (1990)

For grades 7–12. Written by the well-known editor in chief of *Forbes* magazine. Malcolm Forbes and Jeff Block have written brief vignettes of women who have made major contributions in a variety of fields. Some of the women portrayed have significant disabilities.

References

Alberti, R. E., & Emmons, M. L. (1970). *Your perfect right*. San Luis Obispo, CA: Impact.

Alper, S. K., Schloss, P. J., & Schloss, C. N. (1994). *Families of students with disabilities*. Boston: Allyn & Bacon.

American Psychiatric Glossary. (1988). Washington, DC: American Psychiatric Press.

Anderson, W., Chitwood, S., & Hayden, D. (1997). *Negotiating the special education maze: A guide for parents and teachers* (3rd ed.). Bethesda, MD: Woodbine.

Arkava, M. L., & Mueller, D. N. (1976). Components of foster care for handicapped children. *Child Welfare, 58,* 339–345.

Arnold, K. K., Michael, M. G., Hosley, C. A., & Miller, S. (in press). Factors influencing attitudes about family–school communication for parents of children with mild learning problems: Preliminary findings. *Journal of Educational and Psychological Consultation*.

Aspy, D. N. (1969). The effect of teacher-offered conditions of empathy, congruence, and positive regard upon student achievement. *Florida Journal of Educational Research, 11,* 39–48.

Aspy, D. N., & Roebuck, F. N. (1967). An investigation of the relationship between levels of cognitive functioning and the teacher's classroom behavior. *Journal of Educational Research, 8,* 43–48.

Autin, D. (1999, May). Inclusion and the new IDEA. *Exceptional Parent,* pp. 66–70.

Ayers, W. (1986). Thinking about teachers and the curriculum. *Harvard Educational Review, 56,* 49–51.

Bailard, V., & Strang, R. (1964). *Parent–teacher conferences*. New York: McGraw-Hill.

Barnwell, D. A., & Day, M. (1996). Providing support to diverse families. In P. J. Beckman (Ed.), *Strategies for working with families of young children with disabilities* (pp. 47–68). Baltimore: Brookes.

Barsch, R. H. (1968). *The parent of the handicapped child: The study of child-rearing practices*. Springfield, IL: Thomas.

Barsch, R. H. (1969). *The teacher–parent partnership*. Arlington, VA: Council for Exceptional Children.

Bauer, A. M., & Shea, T. M. (1999). *Inclusion 101: How to teach all learners*. Baltimore: Brookes.

Baum, M. H. (1962). Some dynamic factors affecting family adjustment to the handicapped child. *Exceptional Children, 28*, 387–392.

Beckman, P. J. (1983). Influence of selected child characteristics on stress in families of handicapped infants. *American Journal of Mental Deficiency, 88*, 150–156.

Beckman, P. J. (1996). *Strategies for working with families of young children with disabilities*. Baltimore: Brookes.

Beckman, P. J., & Stepanck, J. S. (1996). Facilitating collaboration in meetings and conferences. In P. J. Beckman (Ed.), *Strategies for working with families of young children with disabilities* (pp. 91–107). Baltimore: Brookes.

Benjamin, A. (1974). *The helping interview*. Boston: Houghton Mifflin.

Benjamin, A. (1987). *The helping interview: With case illustrations*. Boston: Houghton Mifflin.

Berger, E. H. (1981). *Parents as partners in education*. New York: Grove Press.

Bergin, A. E. (1963). The effects of psychotherapy. *Journal of Counseling Psychology, 10*, 244–255.

Bernard, A. W. (1974). A comparative study of marital integration and sibling role tension differences between families who have a severely mentally retarded child and families of nonhandicapped (Doctoral dissertation, University of Cincinnati). *Dissertation Abstracts International, 35A*(5), 2800–2801.

Bernheim, K. F., & Lehman, A. (1985). *Working with families of the mentally ill*. New York: Norton.

Berscheid, E., & Walster, E. H. (1969). *Interpersonal attraction*. Reading, MA: Addison-Wesley.

Bibring, G. L., Dwyer, D. S., Huntingdon, D. S., & Vatenstein, A. F. (1961). A study of the psychological processes in pregnancy and the earliest mother–child relationships. *Psychoanalytic Studies of the Child, 16*, 9–72.

Bissell, N. E. (1976). Communicating with the parents of exceptional children. In E. J. Webster (Ed.), *Professional approaches with parents of handicapped children* (pp. 217–229). Springfield, IL: Thomas.

Blacher, J. (1984). *Severely handicapped young children and their families*. Orlando, FL: Academic Press.

Blake, H. E. (1977). *Creating a learning-centered classroom*. New York: Hart.

Bourne, E. J. (1990). *The anxiety and phobia workbook*. Oakland, PA: New Harbinger.

Bowlby, J. (1951). *Maternal care and mental health.* Geneva: World Health Organization.

Bradley, D. F., King-Sears, M., & Tessier-Switlick, D. M. (1997). *Teaching students in inclusive settings.* Boston: Allyn & Bacon.

Brammer, L. M. (1973). *The helping relationship.* Englewood Cliffs, NJ: Prentice-Hall.

Branan, J. M. (1972). Negative human interaction. *Journal of Counseling Psychology, 19,* 81–82.

Brinthaupt, G. (1991). The family of a child with cystic fibrosis. In M. Seligman (Ed.), *The family with a handicapped child* (2nd ed., pp. 295–336). Needham Heights, MA: Allyn & Bacon.

Bristol, M. M. (1984). Family resources and successful adaptation to autistic children. In E. Schopler & G. B. Mesibov (Eds.), *The effects of autism on the family* (pp. 289–310). New York: Plenum.

Bronfenbrenner, U. (1979). *The ecology of human development.* Cambridge, MA: Harvard University Press.

Buriel, R. (1983). Teacher–student interaction and their relationship to student achievement: A comparison of Mexican-American children. *Journal of Educational Psychology, 75,* 889–897.

Buscaglia, L. (1975). *The disabled and their parents: A counseling challenge.* Thorofare, NJ: Slack.

Cantwell, D. P., & Baker, L. (1984). Research concerning families of children with autism. In E. Shopler & A. B. Mesibov (Eds.), *The effects of autism on the family* (pp. 41–63). New York: Plenum.

Carberry, H. (1975). Parent–teacher conferences. *Today's Education, 65,* 67.

Carkhuff, R. R. (1968). Differential functioning of lay and professional helpers. *Journal of Counseling Psychology, 15,* 117–126.

Carkhuff, R. R. (1969). *Helping and human relationships.* New York: Holt, Rinehart & Winston.

Carter, E., & McGoldrick, M. (1980). *The family life cycle.* New York: Gardner.

Chaukin, N. F., & Williams, D. L. (1988). Critical issues in teacher training for parent involvement. *Educational Horizons, 66,* 87–89.

Chesler, M. A., & Barbarin, O. A. (1987). *Childhood cancer and the family.* New York: Brunner/Mazel.

Chigier, E. (1972). *Down's syndrome.* Lexington, MA: Heath.

Click, J. (1986). Grandparent concerns: Learning to be special. *Sibling Information Network Newsletter, 5,* 3–4.

Cohen, K. M., & Kimmerling, F. G. (1971). *Attitudes based on English dialect differences: An analysis of current research* (ED 056 579). Cambridge, MA: Language Research Foundation.

Combs, A. W., Blume, A., Newman, A. J., & Wass, H. L. (1974). *The professional education of teachers.* Boston: Allyn & Bacon.

Corrigan, D. C., & Howey, K. R. (1980). The future: Creating the conditions for professional practice. In D. C. Corrigan & K. R. Howey (Eds.), *Special education in transition* (pp. 268–279). Reston, VA: Council for Exceptional Children.

Council for Exceptional Children. (undated). *Working with parents of exceptional children*. Reston, VA: Council for Exceptional Children.

Crnic, K., Greenberg, N. T., Ragosin, A. S., Robinson, N. M., & Basham, R. B. (1983). Effects of stress and social support on mothers and premature and full-term infants. *Child Development, 54,* 209–217.

Dale, B. (1995). Creating answers. In D. J. Meyer (Ed.), *Uncommon fathers* (pp. 1–12). Bethesda, MD: Woodbine.

Damrosh, S. P., & Perry, L. A. (1989). Self reported adjustment, chronic sorrow, and coping of parents of children with Down syndrome. *Nursing Research, 38,* 25–30.

Darling, R. B. (1979). *Families against society: A study of reactions to children with birth defects*. Beverly Hills, CA: Sage.

Darling, R. B. (1991). Initial and continuing adaptation to the birth of a disabled child. In M. Seligman (Ed.), *The family with a handicapped child* (2nd ed., pp. 55–89). Boston: Allyn & Bacon.

Darling, R. B., & Baxter, C. (1996). *Families in focus: Sociological methods in early intervention*. Austin, TX: Pro-Ed.

Darling, R. B., & Peter, M. I. (1994). *Families, physicians, and children with special health needs: Collaborative medical education models*. Westport, CT: Greenwood.

Davison, G. C., & Neale, J. M. (1990). *Abnormal psychology* (5th ed.). New York: Wiley.

Dawes, R. M. (1994). *House of cards*. New York: Free Press.

Dixon, H. (1995). My inspiration and hope. In D. J. Meyer (Ed.), *Uncommon fathers* (pp. 113–123). Bethesda, MD: Woodbine.

Does therapy help? (1995, November). *Consumer Reports*.

Dorner, S. (1975). The relationship of physical handicap to stress in families with an adolescent with spina bifida. *Developmental Medicine and Child Neurology, 17,* 765–776.

Drotar, D., Baskiewicz, A., Irvin, A., Kennell, J., & Klaus, M. (1975). The adaption of parents to the birth of an infant with congenital malformation: A hypothetical model. *Pediatrics, 56,* 710–717.

Duncan, D. (1977, May). *The impact of a handicapped child upon the family*. Paper presented at the Pennsylvania Training Model Sessions, Harrisburg.

Dushenko, T. (1981). Cystic fibrosis: Medical overview and critique of the psychological literature. *Social Science in Medicine, 15B,* 43–56.

Duvall, E. (1957). *Family development*. Philadelphia: Lippincott.

Egan, G. (1986). *The skilled helper* (3rd ed.). Monterey, CA: Brooks/Cole.

Egan, G. (1990). *The skilled helper* (4th ed.). Pacific Grove, CA: Brooks/Cole.

Egan, G. (1994). *The skilled helper* (5th ed.). Pacific Grove, CA: Brooks/Cole.

Egan, G. (1998). *The skilled helper* (6th ed.). Pacific Grove, CA: Brooks/Cole.

Ekman, P. (1964). Baby position, facial expression, and verbal behavior during interviews. *Journal of Abnormal and Social Psychology, 68,* 295–301.

Elman, N. (1991). Family therapy. In M. Seligman (Ed.), *The family with a handicapped child* (2nd ed., pp. 369–406). Boston: Allyn & Bacon.

Eysenck, H. J. (1955). The effects of psychotherapy: A reply. *Journal of Abnormal Social Psychology, 50,* 147–148.

Falicov, C. J. (1997). "So they don't need me anymore": Weaving migration, illness, and coping. In S. H. McDaniel, J. Hepworth, & W. J. Doherty (Eds.), *The shared experience of illness* (pp. 48–57). New York: Basic Books.

Fanos, J. H. (1996). *Sibling loss.* Mahwah, NJ: Erlbaum.

Farber, B. (1959). Effects of a severely mentally retarded child on family integration. *Monographs of the Society for Research in Child Development, 24*(Serial No. 71).

Farber, B. (1975). Family adaptations to severely mentally retarded children. In M. J. Begab & S. A. Richardson (Eds.), *The mentally retarded child and society: A social science perspective* (pp. 247–266). Baltimore: University Park Press.

Farber, B., & Ryckman, D. B. (1965). Effects of a severely retarded child on family relationships. *Mental Retardation Abstracts, 11,* 1–17.

Featherstone, H. (1980). *A difference in the family.* New York: Basic Books.

Feldman, M. A., Byalick, A. R., & Rosedale, M. P. (1975). Parents and professionals: A partnership in special education. *Exceptional Children, 41,* 551–554.

Fewell, R. (1986). A handicapped child in the family. In R. R. Fewell & P. F. Vadasy (Eds.), *Families of handicapped children* (pp. 3–34). Austin, TX: Pro-Ed.

Fewell, R. R. (1991). Parenting moderately handicapped person. In M. Seligman (Ed.), *The family with a handicapped child* (2nd ed., pp. 203–232). Boston: Allyn & Bacon.

Fine, M. J., & Carlson, C. (1992). *The handbook of family–school intervention: A systems perspective.* Needham Heights, MA: Allyn & Bacon.

Firestein, S. K. (1989). Special features of grief reactions with reproductive catastrophe. *Loss, Grief and Care, 3,* 37–45.

Fox, R. M., Luszki, M., & Schmuck, R. (1966). *Diagnosing classroom learning.* Chicago: SRA.

Freud, A. (1948). *The ego and the mechanisms of defense.* London: Hogarth Press.

Friend, M., & Bursuck, W. D. (1999). *Including students with special needs* (2nd ed.). Needham Heights, MA: Allyn & Bacon.

Gabel, H., McDowell, J., & Cerreto, M. C. (1983). Family adaptation to the handicapped infant. In S. G. Garwood & R. R. Fewell (Eds.), *Educating handicapped infants* (pp. 455–493). Rockville, MD: Aspen.

Gargiulo, R. M. (1985). *Working with parents of exceptional children.* Boston: Houghton Mifflin.

Gillespie, E., & Turnbull, A. P. (1983). Involving special education students on planning the IEP. *Teaching Exceptional Children, 16,* 27–29.

Gilliam, S. K., & Coleman, M. C. (1981). Who influences IEP committee decisions? *Exceptional Children, 47,* 642–644.

Gladding, S. T. (1998). *Family therapy: History, theory and practice.* Upper Saddle River, NJ: Prentice Hall.

Glass, S. D. (1969). *The practical handbook of group counseling.* Baltimore: BCS.

Gorham, K. A., DesJardins, R., Page, E., Pettis, E., & Scheiber, B. (1975). Effects on parents. In N. Hobbs (Ed.), *Issues in the classification of children* (pp. 154–188). San Francisco: Jossey-Bass.

Greenfeld, J. (1978). *A place for Noah*. New York: Pocket Books.

Grossman, F. K. (1972). *Brothers and sisters of retarded children*. Syracuse, NY: Syracuse University Press.

Harris, S. L. (1983). *Families of the developmentally disabled*. New York: Pergamon Press.

Harris, S. L. (1994). *Siblings of children with autism: A guide for families*. Rockville, MD: Woodbine.

Harry, B. (1992). *Cultural diversity, families, and the special education system*. New York: Teachers College Press.

Heaton, J. A. (1998). *Building basic therapeutic skills*. San Francisco: Jossey-Bass.

Henderson, R. W. (1980). Social and emotional needs of culturally diverse children. *Exceptional Children, 46,* 598–605.

Hensie, L. E., & Campbell, R. J. (1970). *Psychiatric dictionary* (4th ed.). London: Oxford University Press.

Herman, R. I. (1983, Fall). Poverty, minority and exceptionality. *Educational Forum,* pp. 47–63.

Hetznecker, W., Arnold, E. L., & Phillips, A. (1978). Teachers, principals and parents. In E. L. Arnold (Ed.), *Helping parents help their children* (pp. 363–376). New York: Brunner/Mazel.

Hill, R. (1949). *Families under stress*. New York: Free Press.

Hobbs, N., Perrin, A., & Ireys, S. (1986). *Chronically ill children and their families*. San Francisco: Jossey-Bass.

Hoge, R. D., & Luce, S. (1979). Predicting academic achievement from classroom behavior. *Review of Educational Research, 49,* 479–496.

Hollingsworth, C. E., & Pasnaw, R. G. (1977). *The family in mourning: A guide for health professionals*. New York: Grune & Stratton.

Hornby, G. (1988). *Fathers of handicapped children*. Unpublished manuscript, University of Hull, UK.

Hornby, G. (1994). *Counseling in child disability*. London: Chapman & Hall.

Hornby, G. (1995). *Working with parents of children with special needs*. London: Cassell.

Hornby, G., & Ashworth, T. (1994). Grandparent support for families who have children with disabilities: A survey of parents. *Journal of Child and Family Studies, 3,* 403–412.

Houser, R., & Seligman, M. (1991). Differences in coping strategies used by fathers of adolescents with disabilities and fathers of adolescents without disabilities. *Journal of Applied Rehabilitation Counseling, 22,* 7–10.

Houston, W. R., & Houston, E. (1992). Needed: A new knowledge base in teacher education. In L. Kaplan (Ed.), *Education and the family* (pp. 255–265). Boston: Allyn & Bacon.

Hymovich, D. P., & Hagopian, G. A. (1992). *Chronic illness in children and adults*. Philadelphia: Saunders.

Imber-Black, E. (1988). *Families and larger systems*. New York: Guilford Press.

Ivey, A. E. (1971). *Microcounseling: Innovations in interviewing.* Springfield, IL: Thomas.

Ivey, A. E. (1983). *Intentional interviewing and counseling.* Monterey, CA: Brooks/Cole.

Ivey, A. E. (1994). *Intentional interviewing and counseling* (3rd ed.). Pacific Grove, CA: Brooks/Cole.

Jackson, G., & Cosca, C. (1974). The inequality of educational opportunities in the Southwest: An observational study of ethnically-mixed classrooms. *American Educational Research Journal, 11,* 219–229.

Jakubowski-Specter, P., Dustin, R., & George, R. (1971). Toward developing a behavioral counselor education model. *Counselor Education and Supervision, 10,* 242–250.

Jessop, D. J., & Stein, R. E. (1985). Uncertainty and its relation to the psychological and social correlates of chronic illness in children. *Social Science and Medicine, 20,* 993–999.

Johnson, D. E., & Vestermark, M. J. (1970). *Barriers and hazards in counseling.* Boston: Houghton Mifflin.

Johnson, E. G., Gerard, H. B., & Miller, N. (1975). Teacher influences in the desegregated classroom: Factors mediating the school desegregation experience. In H. B. Gerard & N. Miller (Eds.), *School desegregation* (pp. 243–259). New York: Plenum.

Kagan, N. I., Holmes, M., & Kagan, H. (Eds.). (1995). *Interpersonal process recall manual.* Houston: Mason Media.

Kahana, G., & Kahana, E. (1970). Grandparenthood from the perspective of the developing grandchild. *Developmental Psychology, 3,* 98–105.

Kalins, I. (1983). Cross-illness comparisons of separation and divorce among parents having a child with a life-threatening illness. *Children's Health Care, 12,* 100–102.

Kaplan, L. (Ed.). (1992). *Education and the family.* Boston: Allyn & Bacon.

Kavanagh, K. H., & Kennedy, P. H. (1992). *Promoting cultural diversity: Strategies for health care professionals.* Newbury Park, CA: Sage.

Kazak, A. E., & Marvin, R. S. (1984). Differences, difficulties and adaption: Stress and social networks in three samples. *Journal of Abnormal Child Psychology, 15,* 137–146.

Kazak, A. E., & Wilcox, B. L. (1984). The structure and function of social support networks in families with handicapped children. *American Journal of Community Psychology, 12,* 645–661.

Khan, S. B., & Weiss, J. (1972). Teaching of affective responses. In R. M. Travers (Ed.), *Second handbook of research on teaching* (pp. 759–804). Chicago: Rand McNally.

Knapp, M. L. (1978). *Nonverbal communication in human interaction* (2nd ed.). New York: Holt, Reinhart, & Winston.

Konopka, G. (1972). *Social group work: A helping process* (2nd ed.). Englewood Cliffs, NJ: Prentice-Hall.

Konstam, V., Drainoni, M., Mitchell, G., Houser, R., Reddington, D., & Eaton, D.

(1993). Career choices and values of sibling of individuals with developmental disabilities. *The School Counselor, 40,* 287–292

Korn, S. J., Chess, S., & Fernandez, P. (1978). The impact of children's physical handicaps on marital quality and family interaction. In R. M. Lerner & G. B. Spanier (Eds.), *Child influences on marital and family interaction: A life-span perspective* (pp. 46–59). New York: Academic Press.

Krahn, G. L. (1993). Conceptualizing social support in families of children with special health needs. *Family Process, 32,* 235–248.

Kroth, R. L. (1975). *Communicating with parents of exceptional children.* Denver: Love.

Kroth, R. L. (1985). *Communicating with parents of exceptional children* (2nd ed.). Denver: Love.

Kroth, R. L., & Edge, D. (1997). *Strategies for communicating with parents and families of exceptional children* (3rd ed.). Denver: Love.

Kübler-Ross, E. (1969). *On death and dying.* New York: Macmillan.

Kundera, M. (1980). *The book of laughter and forgetting.* New York: Penguin.

Kushner, H. S. (1981). *When bad things happen to good people.* New York: Avon Books.

Laborde, R., & Seligman, M. (1983). Counseling parents of children with disabilities: Rationale and strategies. In M. Seligman (Ed.), *The family with a handicapped child* (pp. 337–365). Boston: Allyn & Bacon.

Laborde, P. R., & Seligman, M. (1991). Counseling parents of children with disabilities. In M. Seligman (Ed.), *The family with a handicapped child* (2nd ed., pp. 341–365). Boston: Allyn & Bacon.

Lamb, M. E., & Meyer, D. J. (1991). Fathers of children with special needs. In M. Seligman (Ed.), *The family with a handicapped child* (2nd ed., pp. 151–170). Boston: Allyn & Bacon.

Lambie, R. (2000). *Family systems within educational contexts* (2nd ed.). Denver: Love.

Lambie, R., & Daniels-Mohring, D. (1993). *Family systems within educational contexts: Understanding students with special needs.* Denver: Love.

Laosa, L. M. (1977). Inequality in the classroom. *Aztlan International Journal of Chicano Studies Research, 8,* 51–67.

Lazarus, R., & Folkman, S. (1984). *Stress, appraisal, and coping.* New York: Springer.

Lechtenberg, R. (1984). *Epilepsy and the family.* Cambridge, MA: Harvard University Press.

Lederer, W. J., & Jackson, D. D. (1968). *The mirages of marriage.* New York: Norton.

Leviton, A., Meullen, M., & Kauffmann, C. (1992). The family centered consultation model. *Infants and Young Children, 4,* 1–8.

Lieberman, M. A. (1990). A group therapist perspective on self-help groups. In M. Seligman & L. Marshak (Eds.), *Group psychotherapy: Interventions with special populations* (pp. 1–18). Boston: Allyn & Bacon.

Lightfoot, S. L. (1981). Toward conflict resolution: Relationships between families and schools. *Theory into Practice, 20,* 97–104.

Lisbe, E. R. (1978). Professionals in the public schools. In J. S. Mearig (Ed.), *In working for children* (pp. 239–261). San Francisco: Jossey-Bass.

Lister, J. L. (1966). Counselor experiencing: Its implications for suspervision. *Counselor Educaton and Supervision, 5,* 55–60.

Lobato, D. J. (1990). *Brothers, sisters, and special needs: Information and activities for helping young siblings of children with chronic illnesses and developmental disabilities.* Baltimore: Brookes.

Lombana, J. H. (1983). *Home–school partnerships.* New York: Grune & Stratton.

Lortie, D. C. (1975). *Schoolteacher: A sociological study.* Chicago: University of Chicago Press.

Losen, S., & Diament, B. (1978). *Parent conferences in the schools.* Boston: Allyn & Bacon.

Luszki, M. B., & Schmuck, R. (1965). Pupil perceptions of parental attitudes toward school. *Mental Hygiene, 49,* 296–307.

Luterman, D. (1984). *Counseling the communicatively disordered and their families.* Boston: Little, Brown.

Lynch, E. W. (1992). Developing cross-cultural competence. In E. W. Lynch & M. J. Hanson (Eds.), *Developing cross-cultural competence: A guide for working with young children and their families* (pp. 35–59). Baltimore: Brookes.

Lynch, E. W., & Lewis, R. B. (1988). *Exceptional children and adults.* Glenview, IL: Scott, Foresman.

Lynch, E. W., & Stein, R. (1982). Perspectives on parent participation in special education. *Exceptional Education Quarterly, 3,* 56–63.

Lyon, H. C. (1971). *Learning to feel—feeling to learn.* Columbus, OH: Merrill.

Lyon, S. R., & Lyon, G. (1991). Collaboration with families of persons with severe disabilities. In M. Seligman (Ed.), *The family with a handicapped child* (2nd ed., pp. 237–268). Boston: Allyn & Bacon.

Malmberg, P.A. (1984). *Development of field tested special education placement committee parent education materials.* Unpublished doctoral dissertation, Virginia Polytechnic Institute at State University, Blacksburg.

Marion, R. L. (1992). The mentally retarded child in the family. In M. J. Fine & C. Carlson (Eds.), *The handbook of family–school intervention* (pp. 134–156). Boston: Allyn & Bacon.

Marsh, D. T. (1992). *Families and mental retardation: New directions in professional practice.* New York: Praeger.

Marsh, D. T. (1993). *Families and mental illness.* New York: Praeger.

Marshak, L. E., & Seligman, M. (1993). *Counseling persons with physical disabilities: Theoretical and clinical perspectives.* Austin, TX: Pro-Ed.

Marshak, L. M., Seligman, M., & Prezant, F. (1999). *Disability and the family life cycle: Recognizing and treating developmental challenges.* New York: Basic Books.

Martin, P. (1975). Marital breakdown in families of patients with spina bifida cystica. *Developmental Medicine and Child Neurology, 17,* 757–764.

Max, L. (1985). Parents' views of provisions, services, and research. In N. N. Singh & K. M. Wilton (Eds.), *Mental retardation in New Zealand* (pp. 250–262). Christchurch, New Zealand: Whitcoulls.

McCracken, M. J. (1984). Cystic fibrosis in adolescence. In R. W. Blum (Ed.),

Chronic illness and disability in childhood and adolescence (pp. 397–411). Orlando, FL: Grune & Stratton.

McCubbin, H. I., & Patterson, J. M. (1983). The family stress process: The double ABCX model of adjustment and adaptation. *Marriage and Family Review, 6,* 7–37.

McDaniel, S. H., Hepworth, J., & Doherty, W. J. (1992). *Medical family therapy.* New York: Basic Books.

McGoldrick, M., & Giordano, J. (1996). Overview: Ethnicity and family therapy. In M. McGoldrick, J. Giordano, & J. K. Pearce (Eds.), *Ethnicity and family therapy* (2nd ed., pp. 1–27). New York: Guilford Press.

McGoldrick, M., Giordano, J., & Pearce, J. K. (Eds.). (1996). *Ethnicity and family therapy* (2nd ed.). New York: Guilford Press.

McHugh, M. (1999). *Special siblings: Growing up with someone with a disability.* New York: Hyperion.

McKay, M., & Fanning, P. (1997). *The daily relaxer.* Oakland, PA: New Harbinger.

McPhee, N. (1982, June). A very special magic: A grandparents delight. *Exceptional Parents, 12,* 13–16.

Mehrabian, A. (1971). *Silent messages.* Belmont, CA: Wadsworth.

Meyan, E. L., Vergason, G. A., & Whelan, R. J. (1996). *Strategies for teaching exceptional children in inclusive settings.* Denver: Love.

Meyer, D. J. (1995). *Uncommon fathers: Reflections on raising a child with a disability.* Bethesda, MD: Woodbine.

Meyer, D. J., & Vadasy, P. F. (1986). *Grandparent workshops: How to organize workshops for grandparents of children with handicaps.* Seattle: University of Washington Press.

Meyer, D. J., & Vadasy, P. F. (1994). *Sibships: Workshops for siblings of children with special needs.* Baltimore: Brookes.

Meyer, D. J., Vadasy, P. F., Fewell, R. R., & Schell, G. C. (1985). *A handbook for the fathers program.* Seattle: University of Washington Press.

Minkler, M., & Roe, K. M. (1993). *Grandparents as caregivers: Raising the children of the crack cocaine epidemic.* Thousand Oaks, CA: Sage.

Minuchin, S. (1974). *Psychosomatic families.* Cambridge, MA: Harvard University Press.

Moeller, C. J. (1986). The effect of professionals on the family of a handicapped child. In R. R. Fewell & P. F. Vadasy (Eds.), *Families of handicapped children* (pp. 149–166). Austin, TX: Pro-Ed.

Moorman, M. (1992, January/February). My sister's keeper. *Family Therapy Networker,* pp. 41–47.

Moos, R. H. (1984). *Coping with physical illness.* New York: Plenum.

Mullins, J. (1979). *A teacher's guide to management of physically handicapped students.* Springfield, IL: Thomas.

Murphy, B. C., & Dillon, C. (1998). *Interviewing in action: Process and practice.* Pacific Grove, CA: Brooks/Cole.

Napier, R. W., & Gershenfeld, M. K. (1981). *Groups: Theory and experience.* Boston: Houghton Mifflin.

Napier, R. W., & Gershenfeld, M. K. (1999). *Groups: Theory and experience* (5th ed.). Boston: Houghton Mifflin.

Naseef, R. A. (1997). *Special children, challenged parents*. Secaucus, NJ: Birch Lane Press.

Neugarten, B. L. (1976). Adaptation and the life cycle. *Counseling Psychologist, 6*, 16–20.

Neugeboren, J. (1997). *Imagining Robert: My brother, madness, and survival*. New York: Morrow.

Nichols, M. P. (1995). *The lost art of listening*. New York: Guilford Press.

Noble, L. S., & Euster, S. D. (1981). Foster parent input: A crucial element in training. *Child Welfare, 60*, 35–42.

Offer, D., Ostrov, E., & Howard, K. I. (1984). Body image, self-perception, and chronic illness in adolescence. In R. W. Blum (Ed.), *Chronic illness and disability in childhood and adolescence* (pp. 59–73). Orlando, FL: Grune & Stratton.

O'Halloran, J. M. (1993). Welcome to our family, Casey Patrick. In A. P. Turnbull, J. M. Patterson, S. K. Behr, D. L. Murphy, J. G. Marquis, & M. J. Blue-Banning (Eds.), *Cognitive coping, families, and society* (pp. 19–29). Baltimore: Brookes.

Olshansky, S. (1962). Chronic sorrow: A response to having a mentally defective child. *Social Casework, 43*, 190–193.

Olson, D. H., McCubbin, H. I., Barnes, H., Larsen, H., Muxen, M., & Wilson, M. (1984). *One thousand families: A national survey*. Beverly Hills, CA: Sage.

Olson, D. H., Russell, C. S., & Sprenkle, D. H. (1980). Circumplex Model of Marital and Family Systems II. In J. P. Vincent (Ed.), *Advances in family intervention assessment and theory* (Vol. 7, pp. 129–179). Greenwich, CT: JAI Press.

Pagel, S., & Price, J. (1980). Strategies to alleviate teacher stress. *Pointer, 24*, 45–53.

Palomares, G. D. (1970). *The effects of stereotyping on the self-concept of Mexican-Americans* (ED 056 806). Albuquerque, NM: Southwestern Cooperative Educational Laboratory.

Parke, R. D. (1981). *Fathers*. Cambridge, MA: Harvard University Press.

Patterson, J. M. (1985). Critical factors affecting family compliance with home treatment for children with cystic fibrosis. *Family Relations, 34*, 79–89.

Patterson, J. M. (1988). Chronic illness in children and the impact on families. In C. S. Chilmon, E. W. Nunnally, & F. M. Cox (Eds.), *Chronic illness and disabilities* (pp. 69–107). Beverly Hills, CA: Sage.

Patterson, J. M. (1991). A family systems perspective for working with youth with disabilities. *Pediatrician, 18*, 129–141.

Peck, J. R., & Stephens, W. B. (1960). A study of the relationship between the attitudes and behavior of parents and that of their mentally defective child. *American Journal of Mental Deficiency, 64*, 839–844.

Perrin, J., & MacLean, W. E. (1988). Biomedical and psychosocial dimensions of chronic illness in childhood. In P. Kardy (Ed.), *Handbook of child health assessment* (pp. 111–129). New York: Wiley.

Peterson, J. V., & Nisenholz, B. (1987). *Orientation to counseling*. Boston: Allyn & Bacon.

Petr, C. G., & Barney, D. D. (1993). Reasonable efforts for children with disabilities: The parents' perspective. *Social Work, 38*, 247–254.

Pieper, E. (1976, April). Grandparents can help. *Exceptional Parent*, pp. 7–9.

Pistono, U. J. (1977). The relationship between certain identified variables and parent participation during the Educational Planning and Placement Committee Meeting for handicapped students in Michigan. *Dissertation Abstracts International, 38*(5A), 2705.

Pittsburgh Post Gazette. (1998, August 3). p. A–6.

Powell, T. H., & Gallagher, P. A. (1993). *Brothers and sisters: A special part of exceptional families* (2nd ed.). Baltimore: Brookes.

Pruett, K. D. (1987). *The nurturing father.* New York: Warner.

Ramsey, C. N., Jr. (Ed). (1989). *Family systems in medicine.* New York: Guilford Press.

Raven, B. H., & Rubin, J. Z. (1976). *Social psychology.* New York: Wiley.

Reik, T. (1972). *Listening with the third ear.* New York: Farrar, Straus & Giroux.

Reynolds, M. C., & Birch, J. W. (1977). *Teaching exceptional children in all America's schools.* Reston, VA: Council for Exceptional Children.

Reynolds, M. C., Birch, J. W., Grohs, D., Howsam, R., & Morsink, C. (1980). *A common body of practice for teachers: The challenge of Public Law 94–142 to teacher education.* Washington, DC: American Association of Colleges for Teacher Education.

Rolland, J. S. (1993). Mastering family challenges in serious illness and disability. In F. Walsh (Ed.), *Normal family processes* (2nd ed., pp. 444–473). New York: Guilford Press.

Ross, A. E. (1964). *The exceptional child in the family.* New York: Grune & Stratton.

Rowe, M. (1978). Psychoanalytic insights for parent guidance. In L. E. Arnold (Ed.), *Helping parents help their children* (pp. 37–45). New York: Brunner/Mazel.

Rubin, S., & Quinn-Curran, N. (1983). Lost then found: Parents' journey through the community service maze. In M. Seligman (Ed.), *The family with a handicapped child* (pp. 63–94). Orlando, FL: Grune & Stratton.

Rubin, Z. (1973). *Liking and loving.* New York: Holt, Rinehart & Winston.

Rutherford, R. B., & Edgar, E. (1979). *Teachers and parents: A guide to interaction and cooperation.* Boston: Allyn & Bacon.

Sabbeth, B. F., & Leventhal, J. M. (1984). Marital adjustment to chronic childhood illness: A critique of the literature. *Pediatrics, 73*, 762–768.

Schopler, E., & Mesibov, G. (1984). Professional attitudes toward parents: A forty-year progress report. In E. Schopler & G. B. Mesibov (Eds.), *The effects of autism on the family* (pp. 3–17). New York: Plenum.

Schorr-Ribera, H. K. (1987). *Ethnicity and culture as relevant rehabilitation factors in families with children with disabilities.* Unpublished manuscript, University of Pittsburgh.

Schulman, E. D. (1974). *Intervention in human services.* St. Louis, MO: Mosby.

Schulman, E. D. (1978). *Intervention in human services* (2nd ed.). St. Louis, MO: Mosby.

Schulz, J. B. (1987). *Parents and professionals in special education.* Boston: Allyn & Bacon.

Schwab, L. O. (1989). Strengths of families having a member with a disability. *Journal of Multihandicapped Persons, 2*, 105–117.

Searle, S. J. (1978). Stages of parents reactions. *Exceptional Parent, 8,* 27–29.

Seligman, M. (1979). *Strategies for helping parents of exceptional children.* New York: Free Press.

Seligman, M. (1991a). *The family with a handicapped child* (2nd ed.). Boston: Allyn & Bacon.

Seligman, M. (1991b). Grandparents of disabled children: Hopes, fears, and adaptation. *Families in Society, 72,* 147–152.

Seligman, M. (1993). Group work with children with disabilities. *Journal for Specialists in Group Work, 18,* 115–126.

Seligman, M., & Darling, R. B. (1997). *Ordinary families, special children: A systems approach to childhood disability* (2nd ed.). New York: Guilford Press.

Seligman, M., & Seligman, P. A. (1980). The professional's dilemma: Learning to work with parents. *Exceptional Parent, 10,* 511–513.

Seligman, M. E. P. (1995). The effectiveness of psychotherapy. *American Psychologist, 50,* 965–974.

Seligman, M. E. P., & Rosenhan, D. L. (1998). *Abnormality.* New York: Norton.

Shapiro, L. J. (1975). Teachers and schools, don't be afraid—parents love you. *Journal of Teacher Education, 26,* 269–273.

Shea, T. M., & Bauer, A. M. (1991). *Parents and teachers of children with exceptionalities.* Needham Heights, MA: Allyn & Bacon.

Siegel, B. (1996). *The world of the autistic child.* New York: Oxford.

Siegel, B., & Silverstein, S. (1994). *What about me? Growing up with a developmentally disabled sibling.* New York: Plenum.

Simpson, R. L. (1990). *Conferencing parents of exceptional children.* Austin, TX: Pro-Ed.

Simpson, R. L. (1996). *Working with parents and families of exceptional children and youth* (2nd ed.). Austin, TX: Pro-Ed.

Simpson, R. L., & Fiedler, C. R. (1989). Parent participation in Individualized Educational Program (IEP) conferences. In M. Fine (Ed.), *The second handbook on parent educations: Contemporary perspectives* (pp. 145–171). New York: Academic Press.

Simpson, R. L., & Kamps, D. W. (1996). Exceptional children in today's schools. In E. L. Meyer (Ed.). *Exceptional children in today's school* (3rd ed., pp. 195–212). Denver: Love.

Sloman, M. D., Springer, S., & Vachon, M. (1993). Disordered communication and grieving in deaf member families. *Family Process, 32,* 171–181.

Smith, J. (1979). The education of Mexican-Americans. *Teacher Education and Special Education, 2,* 37–48.

Smith, J., & Cline, D. (1980). Quality programs. *Pointer, 24,* 80–87.

Smith, K. (1981). The influence of the male sex role on discussion groups for fathers of exceptional children. *Michigan Personnel and Guidance Journal, 12,* 11–17.

Solnit, A. J., & Stark, M. H. (1961). Mourning and the birth of a defective child. *Psychoanalytic Study of the Child, 16,* 523–537.

Sommers-Flanagan, J., & Sommers-Flanagan, R. (1993). *Foundations of therapeutic interviewing.* Needham Heights, MA: Allyn & Bacon.

Sonnenschein, P. (1981). Parents and professionals: An uneasy relationship. *Teaching Exceptional Children, 114,* 62–65.

Sourkes, B. M. (1982). *The deepening shade.* Pittsburgh: University of Pittsburgh Press.

Spiegel, J. P. (1957). The resolution of role conflict within the family. *Psychiatry, 20,* 1–16.

Stein, R. E., & Jessop, D. J. (1984). General issues in the care of children with chronic physical conditions. *Pediatric Clinics of North America, 31,* 189–198.

Stern, C., & Keislar, E. R. (1977). Teacher attitudes and attitude change: A research review. *Journal of Research and Development in Education, 10,* 63–75.

Stoneman, Z., & Berman, P. W. (1993). *The effects of mental retardation, disability, and illness on sibling relationships.* Baltimore: Brookes.

Swick, K. J., & Lamb, M. L. (1972). *Development of positive racial attitudes, knowledge, and activities in perspective social studies teachers* (ED 073 025). College of Education, Southern Illinois University, Carbondale, IL.

Tallman, I. (1965). Spousal role differentiation and the socialization of severely retarded children. *Journal of Marriage and the Family, 27,* 37–42.

Tartar, S. B. (1987). *Traumatic head injury: Parental stress, coping style and emotional adjustment.* Unpublished doctoral dissertation, University of Pittsburgh, PA.

Taylor, F. C. (1976). Project cope. In E. J. Webster (Ed.), *Professional approaches with parents of handicapped children* (pp. 341–358). Springfield, IL: Thomas.

Thompson, R. J., & Gustafson, K. E. (1996). *Adaptation to chronic childhood illness.* Washington, DC: American Psychological Association.

Thompson, T. M. (1982). An investigation and comparsion of public school personnel's perception and intergeratation of P.L. 94-142. *Dissertation Abstracts International, 43,* 2840A.

Trainer, M. (1991). *Differences in common.* Rockville, MD: Woodbine.

Travis, C. (1976). *Chronic illness in children: Its impact on child and family.* Stanford, CA: Stanford University Press.

Trueba, H., Jacobs, L., & Kirton, E. (1990). *Cultural conflict and adaptation: The case of Hmong children in American society.* New York: Falmer.

Turk, D. C., & Kerns, R. D. (1985). *Health, illness, and families.* New York: Wiley.

Turnbull, A. P. (1983). Parent–professional interactions. In M. E. Snell (Ed.), *Systematic instruction of the moderately and severely handicapped* (pp. 263–284). Columbus, OH: Merrill.

Turnbull, A. P., Brotherson, M. J., & Summers, J. A. (1985). The impact of deinstitutionalization on families. In R. H. Bruininks (Ed.), *Living and learning in the least restrictive environment* (pp. 115–152). Baltimore: Brookes.

Turnbull, A. P., Patterson, J. M., Behr, S. K., Murphy, D. L., Marquis, J. G., & Blue-Banning, M. J. (1993). *Cognitive coping, families, and disability.* Baltimore: Brookes.

Turnbull, A. P., Summers, J. A., & Brotherson, M. J. (1984). *Working with families with disabled members: A family systems approach.* Lawrence: University of Kansas, Kansas University Affiliated Facility.

Turnbull, A. P., & Turnbull, H. R. (1986). *Families, professionals, and exceptionality: A special partnership.* Columbus, OH: Merrill.

Turnbull, A. P., Turnbull, H. R., Shank, M., & Leal, D. (1995). *Exceptional lives: Special education in today's schools.* Upper Saddle River, NJ: Merrill.

Turnbull, H. R., & Turnbull, A. P. (1985). *Parents speak out.* Columbus, OH: Merrill.

Turner, R. H. (1970). *Family interaction.* New York: Wiley.

Upshur, C. C. (1991). Families and the community service MAZE. In M. Seligman (Ed.), *The family with an handicapped child* (pp. 91–114). Boston: Allyn & Bacon.

Vadasy, P. F. (1986). Single mothers: A social phenomenon and population in need. In R. R. Favell & P. F. Vadasy (Eds.), *Families of handicapped children* (pp. 132–148). Austin, TX: Pro-Ed.

Vadasy, P. F., Fewell, R. R., Greenberg, M. T., Desmond, N. L., & Meyer, D. J. (1986). Follow-up evaluation of the effects of involvement in the fathers program. *Topics in Early Childhood Education, 6,* 16–31.

Vadasy, P. F., Fewell, R. R., & Meyer, D. J. (1986). Grandparents of children with special needs: Insights into their experiences and concerns. *Journal of the Division for Early Childhood Education, 10,* 36–44.

Vadasy, P. F., Fewell, R. R., Meyer, D. J., & Greenberg, M. T. (1985). Supporting fathers of handicapped young children: Preliminary findings of program effects. *Analysis and Intervention in Developmental Disabilities, 5,* 123–137.

Varekamp, M. A., Suurmeijer, P., Rosendaal, F. R., Dijck, H., Uriends, A., & Briet, E. (1990). Family burden in families with a hemophilic child. *Family Systems Medicine, 8,* 291–301.

Venter, M. (1980). *Chronic childhood illness and familial coping.* Unpublished doctoral dissertation, University of Minnesota, Minneapolis, MN.

Visher, E. B., & Visher, J. S. (1988). *How to win as a stepfamily.* New York: Brunner/Mazel.

von Bertalanffy, L. (1968). *General systems theory.* New York: Braziller.

Waisbren, S. E. (1980). Parents' reactions after the birth of a developmentally disabled child. *American Journal of Mental Deficiency, 84,* 345–351.

Wallinga, C., Paquio, L., & Skeen, P. (1987). When a brother or sister is ill. *Psychology Today, 42,* 43.

Walsh, F. (1989). The family in later life. In B. Carter & M. McGoldrick (Eds.), *The changing family life cycle* (2nd ed., pp. 379–402). Needham Heights, MA: Allyn & Bacon.

Walsh, F. (Ed.). (1993). *Normal family processes* (2nd ed.). New York: Guilford Press.

Whiston, S. C., & Sexton, T. L. (1993). An overview of psychotherapy outcome research: Implications for practice. *Professional Psychology: Research and Practice, 24,* 43–51.

Wikler, L. (1981). Chronic stresses of families of mentally retarded children. *Family Relations, 30,* 281–288.

Wikler, L., Wasow, M., & Hatfield, E. (1981). Chronic sorrow revisited. *American Journal of Orthopsychiatry, 51,* 63–70.

Williams, F., Whitehead, J. L., & Miller, L. M. (1971). *Attitudinal correlates of children's speech characteristics* (ED 052 213). Austin, TX: Center for Communication Research, University of Texas.

Witt, J. C., Miller, C. D., McIntyre, R. M., & Smith, D. (1984). Effects of variables on parental perceptions of staffings. *Exceptional Children, 51,* 27–32.

Wittmer, J. (1971). *The school survey of interpersonal relationships.* Linden, NJ: Remediation Associates.

Wittmer, J., & Myrick, R. D. (1974). *Facilitative teaching.* Pacific Palisades, CA: Goodyear.

Wortis, H. Z., & Margolies, J. A. (1955). Parents of children with cerebral palsy. *Medical Social Work, 4,* 110–120.

Yalom, I. (1980). *Existential psychotherapy.* New York: Basic Books.

Yalom, I. (1985). *The theory and practice of group psychotherapy* (3rd ed.). New York: Basic Books.

Yalom, I. (1995). *The theory and practice of group psychotherapy* (4th ed.). New York: Basic Books.

Yalom, I. D., & Lieberman, M. A. (1971). A study of encounter group casualties. *Archives of General Psychiatry, 25,* 16–30.

Zach, L., & Price, M. (1973). *The teacher's part in sex role reinforcement* (ED 070 513). Research in Education.

Index

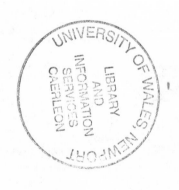